Complex Primary and Revision
Total Knee Arthroplasty

Bryan D. Springer • Brian M. Curtin
Editors

Complex Primary and Revision Total Knee Arthroplasty

A Clinical Casebook

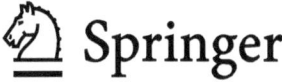 Springer

Editors
Bryan D. Springer, MD
Fellowship Director
OrthoCarolina Hip and Knee
   Center
Charlotte, NC, USA

Brian M. Curtin, MD, MS
OrthoCarolina Hip and Knee
   Center
Charlotte, NC, USA

ISBN 978-3-319-18349-7   ISBN 978-3-319-18350-3   (eBook)
DOI 10.1007/978-3-319-18350-3

Library of Congress Control Number: 2015941446

Springer Cham Heidelberg New York Dordrecht London
© Springer International Publishing Switzerland 2015

Printed on acid-free paper

Springer International Publishing AG Switzerland is part of Springer Science+Business Media (www.springer.com)

Preface

Adult reconstructive surgery of the knee continues to advance at a hectic pace with rapid change in our understanding of the knee. The goal of *Complex Primary and Revision Total Knee Arthroplasty: A Clinical Casebook* is to provide the practicing orthopedic surgeon, fellow, and resident with a concise volume that illustrates much of the basics and multitude of options available to treat both simple and complex adult reconstructive problems. It provides a framework for understanding how to evaluate, diagnose, and treat these problems. The chapters not only provide information on preferred treatments but also summarize many of the latest studies and controversies regarding management and treatment.

Chapter topics were chosen to cover the most pertinent and prevalent areas that a practicing surgeon may encounter. Each chapter is formatted such that the reader can identify a suspected problem and gain additional understanding of the fundamentals that lead to the given situation as well as appropriate management strategies. Chapter authors were selected by the editors for their known expertise in the given subject field and asked to provide real-world case examples to help illustrate the chapter focus. The book is not intended to be a comprehensive and exhaustive consolidation of the most recent and past literature or cover every aspect of each subject. For those readers using the text on an occasional basis to provide deeper understanding or refreshing memory, the chapters are organized concisely and include clinical pearls at the end of each chapter to help reinforce key points and learning objectives. For those reading the book from start to finish, a firm understanding of the essentials and overview of controversial topics may be gained with clinical examples to help with reinforcement and overall learning.

We hope this casebook becomes a frequently referenced companion for the practicing orthopedic surgeon as well as those residents and fellows learning the art of primary and revision knee arthroplasty.

Charlotte, NC, USA   Bryan D. Springer, MD
                                                     Brian M. Curtin, MD, MS

Contents

Contributors

Lucas A. Anderson, MD University of Utah, Salt Lake City, UT, USA

Lucas Armstrong, MD McLean County Orthopedics, Ltd., Bloomington, IL, USA

John W. Barrington, MD Joint Replacement Center of Texas, and Plano Orthopedics and Sports Medicine, Plano, TX, USA

Brian M. Curtin, MD, MS OrthoCarolina Hip and Knee Center, Charlotte, NC, USA

Craig J. Della Valle, MD Rush University Medical Center, Chicago, IL, USA

Brian Evans, MD Department of Orthopedic Surgery, Medstar Georgetown University Hospital, Washington, DC, USA

Jeremy M. Gililland, MD University of Utah, Salt Lake City, UT, USA

Robert G.W. Girling V, MD Department of Orthopedic Surgery, University of Texas Health Science Center at San Antonio, San Antonio, TX, USA

Miguel M. Gomez, MD The Rothman Institute at Thomas Jefferson University, Philadelphia, PA, USA

Raúl G. Gösthe, MD Orthopedic Surgery, Jackson Memorial Hospital, University of Miami, Miami, FL, USA

William A. Jiranek, MD Department of Orthopedic Surgery, VCU Health System, Richmond, VA, USA

Erdan Kayupov, MSE Rush University Medical Center, Chicago, IL, USA

Jorge Manrique, MD The Rothman Institute at Thomas Jefferson University, Philadelphia, PA, USA

Robert M. Molloy, MD Department of Orthopedic Surgery, Cleveland Clinic, Cleveland, OH, USA

Matthew C. Morrey, MD Department of Orthopedic Surgery, University of Texas Health Science Center at San Antonio, San Antonio, TX, USA

Colin A. Mudrick, MD OrthoCarolina Hip and Knee Center, Charlotte, NC, USA

Ryan M. Nunley, BA, MD Department of Orthopedic Surgery, Washington University School of Medicine, St. Louis, MO, USA

Javad Parvizi, MD, FRCS The Rothman Institute at Thomas Jefferson University, Philadelphia, PA, USA

Colin T. Penrose, BS, BA Duke University School of Medicine, Durham, NC, USA

Gregory G. Polkowski, MD, MSc Department of Orthopedic Surgery, Vanderbilt University Medical Center, Nashville, TN, USA

Matthew Russo, MD Department of Orthopedic Surgery, Medstar Georgetown University Hospital, Washington, DC, USA

Bryan D. Springer, MD OrthoCarolina Hip and Knee Center, Charlotte, NC, USA

Juan C. Suarez, MD Orthopedic and Rheumatologic Institute, Cleveland Clinic Florida, Weston, FL, USA

Nicholas T. Ting, MD Department of Orthopedic Surgery, Cleveland Clinic, Cleveland, OH, USA

Clint Wooten, MD OrthoCarolina Hip and Knee Center, Charlotte, NC, USA

Jon O. Wright, BS Department of Orthopedic Surgery, Washington University School of Medicine, St. Louis, MO, USA

Chapter 1
Complex Primary Total Knee Arthroplasty: Management of Varus Knee

Colin T. Penrose and John W. Barrington

1.1 Case Presentation

A 65-year-old male presented to an orthopedic clinic with knee pain along the medial aspect of both knees with the right significantly worse than the left. The patient described frequent morning pain and stiffness, which generally diminished within 15 min; the pain became worse later in the day, especially with significant walking. He sought pain relief with acetaminophen and ibuprofen, but noticed decreasing effectiveness over the last several years. He denied recent trauma, although he reported having minor sports injuries in the distant past. Walking down stairs exacerbated the pain. He was no longer able to jog so he tried to use the elliptical machine for exercise and weight loss, but recently his knee pain prevented him from doing much at all. As a result, he gained 15 lb and his BMI increased to 32. Past medical history included prehypertension but the patient is otherwise in good health.

C.T. Penrose, BS, BA
Duke University School of Medicine, Durham, NC, USA

J.W. Barrington, MD (✉)
Joint Replacement Center of Texas, and Plano Orthopedics and Sports Medicine, Plano, TX, USA
e-mail: jbarrington@sbcglobal.net

© Springer International Publishing Switzerland 2015   1
B.D. Springer and B.M. Curtin (eds.), *Complex Primary and Revision Total Knee Arthroplasty: A Clinical Casebook*, DOI 10.1007/978-3-319-18350-3_1

On physical examination, the patient walked with a slow, bow-legged gait and favored his right leg with a moderate limp. On palpation, pain was elicited along the medial joint line and there was a small effusion with no appreciable warmth. The right knee had a range of motion from 0° to 110° and crepitus was noted. The patient had a correctable varus deformity and no evidence of gross ligamentous instability on Lachman, posterior drawer, or anterior drawer testing.

Plain film radiography revealed advanced arthritic changes with medial joint space narrowing (see Fig. 1.1). The joint space of the lateral compartment was full thickness. There were osteophytes present along the medial distal femur and proximal tibia (see Figs. 1.1 and 1.2). Full-length standing AP views were obtained for preoperative planning (see Fig. 1.3). Sunrise view demonstrated no evidence of pathology at the patellofemoral joint.

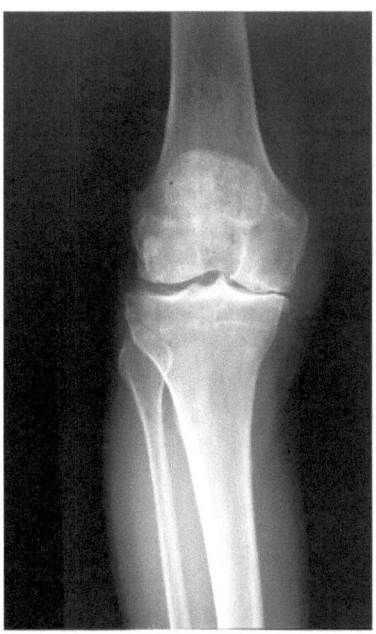

FIG. 1.1. Weight-bearing AP radiograph of the right knee of a 65-year-old male with medial joint space narrowing, osteophytes, and varus deformity.

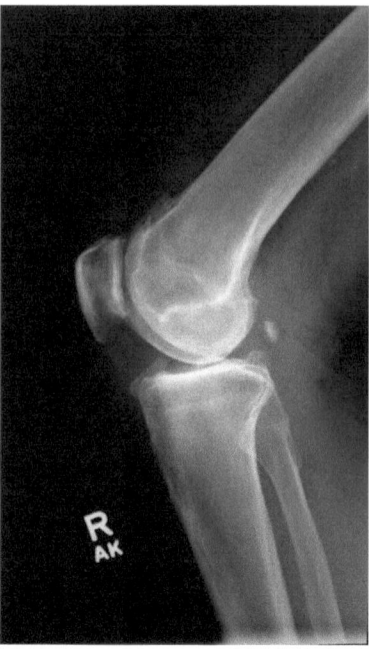

Fig. 1.2. Lateral view radiograph of the right knee of a 65-year-old male.

1.2   Diagnosis/Assessment

Diagnosis of osteoarthritis begins with history and physical exam. Alignment of the knee must be evaluated with physical exam and radiographs. Valgus stress views are useful to confirm full thickness intact lateral cartilage and varus stress views can confirm complete joint space loss medially. A standing PA 45°, or "notch" view, can help distinguish a normal lateral compartment from one with joint pathology (see Fig. 1.4). Severity of varus deformity should be determined preoperatively. It is very important to distinguish a fixed varus deformity from one that is flexible or correctable. Loss of medial joint space can create a pseudolaxity, which

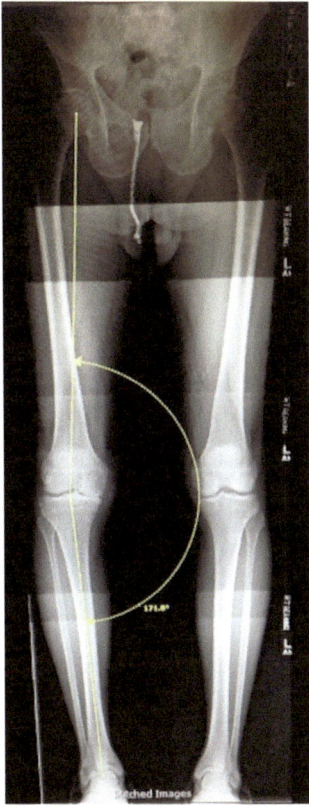

Fɪɢ. 1.3. Full-length radiograph obtained by stitching images together allows accurate measurement of varus deformity and is an important preoperative view to obtain. The comparison to the patient's relatively normal contralateral (*left*) knee highlights the loss of medial cartilage and varus deformity of the right knee.

may lead to overstripping of the MCL during exposure [1]. A full-length x-ray of the lower extremity in both the anterior/posterior and lateral dimensions is often obtained and may be helpful especially in unusual cases (see Fig. 1.3). It is of great importance that the projection is obtained in neutral rotation.

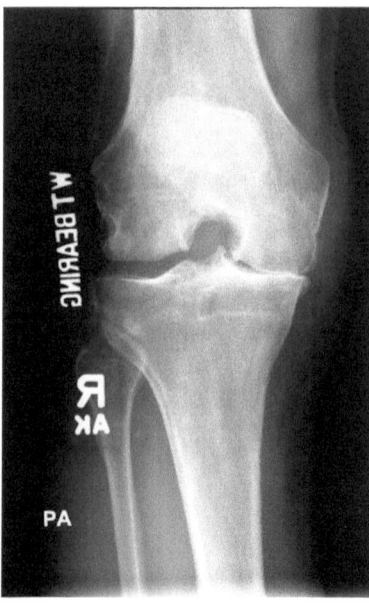

Fig. 1.4. Standing PA 45° ("notch" view) reveals a normal lateral compartment. This is an important criterion to fulfill to consider a unicompartmental knee arthroplasty. If there was pathology in the lateral compartment, this view would cause the lateral compartment to appear collapsed.

1.3 Management

Management of the varus knee may begin conservatively with oral medication, activity modification, weight loss, and unloader bracing. These efforts may allow the patient to function with a reasonable level of pain control and delay the need for more invasive therapies. As the condition continues to progress, there is a role for glucocorticoid injections, which typically provide a temporary therapeutic benefit in addition to diagnostic value when the pain is relieved by targeted injection. Gel injectables (including synvisc and supartz) are also often administered. When these more conservative modalities fail, patients and providers should consider surgical intervention.

1.4   Outcome

After presurgical evaluation and consent for surgery, the patient in this case presentation underwent medial unicompartmental arthroplasty. The patient began walking within hours after the operation. After 3 weeks of rehabilitation with physical therapy and home exercises, the patient had pain-free range of motion from 2° to 110° with good alignment. At 1 year follow-up visit, the patient was doing well clinically. Radiographs revealed good alignment with no evidence of osteolysis (see Figs. 1.5, 1.6, and 1.7).

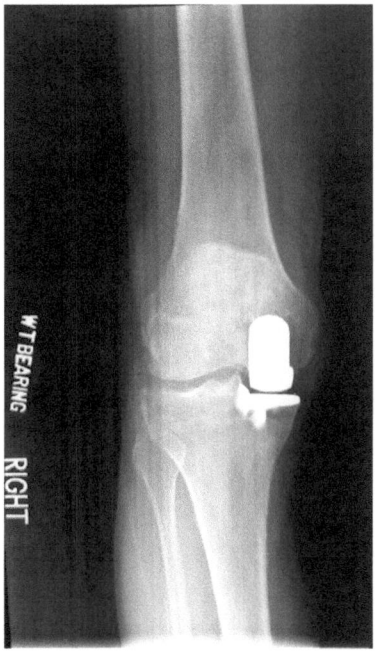

FIG. 1.5. One-year postoperative AP, weight-bearing radiograph of the patient's right knee revealing good alignment of the unicompartmental knee arthroplasty.

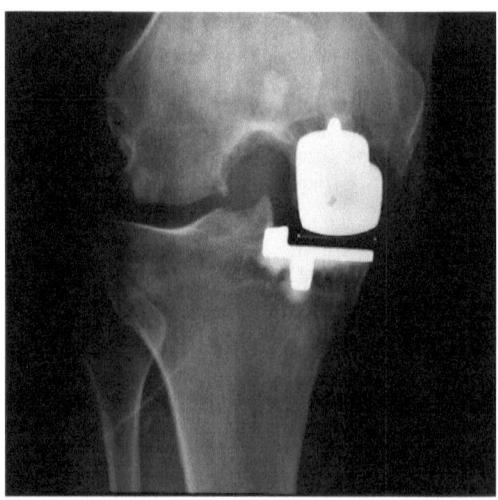

Fig. 1.6. One-year postoperative PA radiograph of the right knee revealing persistent full thickness joint space of the lateral compartment.

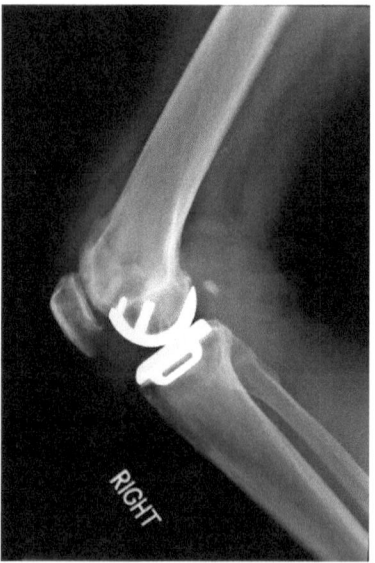

Fig. 1.7. One-year postoperative lateral radiograph of the right knee obtained in flexion.

1.5   Literature Review

Treatment of varus knee after failure of conservative management has been approached in a variety of ways: proximal tibial osteotomy, medial unicompartmental knee arthroplasty, and total knee arthroplasty. Total knee arthroplasty design construct options include ACL and/or PCL sparing, posterior stabilized, constrained, and rotating hinge.

1.5.1   Proximal Tibial Osteotomy

The proximal tibial osteotomy can be effective in shifting the weight-bearing stresses from the medial to the lateral compartment; however, results are much less immediate than with total knee arthroplasty often taking 6 months for recovery. A meta-analysis demonstrated a good or excellent result at 60 months occurred in 75.3 % of cases, and at 100 months in 60.3 % of cases. Based on these results, the authors suggested that in young patients with specific indications, there is a role for closing wedge tibial osteotomy [2]. However, given the long time frame for recovery and less favorable outcomes (as well as improvements in unicompartmental and total knee arthroplasty), this is a less common surgery, primarily reserved for the young, heavy laborer.

1.5.2   Unicompartmental Knee Arthroplasty

Unicompartmental knee arthroplasty is an important operation to consider in varus knee deformity patients with osteoarthritis affecting only the medial compartment. Patients should fulfill the three Carr Criteria to be considered for unicompartmental knee arthroplasty: a functional ACL, fully correctable deformity, and full thickness of lateral compartment articular cartilage [3]. Several large studies have demonstrated excellent results when patients fulfilling these criteria were selected [4, 5]. Obesity has been reported as another contraindication [6]. Unicompartmental knee arthroplasty has been associated with shorter lengths of stay and lower perioperative complications from this less-invasive procedure, although higher revision rates have been associated with this technique when nationwide databases are analyzed [7].

1.5.3   Total Knee Arthroplasty

Varus deformed knees with anterior cruciate ligamentous instability, wear of the cartilage of the lateral compartment, or a deformity that is not fully correctable with valgus stress are best treated with total knee arthroplasty. Rotational alignment of the femoral component is crucial, and the AP axis and epicondylar axis are useful anatomic landmarks to allow balancing of the knee without the need for excessive ligamentous release [8]. When release is required to balance the varus knee, the order in which structures are released is important. The deep medial collateral ligament should be released from the tibia to the posteromedial corner of the knee as part of the initial exposure. All osteophytes from the distal femur and proximal tibia should be removed next because their presence can have a tenting effect on the medial soft tissue sleeve. If a medial contracture remains present, then release should proceed sequentially with the semimembranosus aponeurosis followed by the superficial medial collateral ligament and finally the pes anserinus insertions. Before each of these releases, stability should be assessed to determine the need to proceed. If medial contracture persists and the PCL has been preserved, release of the PCL and careful removal of the posteromedial capsule are indicated with conversion to a PCL-substituting prosthesis. Occasionally, severe medial contracture will require an additional step: stripping the periosteum of the tibia distally 5 cm and fractionally severing the periosteum. It is important to proceed in this order and only after stability has been checked because overrelease leads to valgus instability [9]. Soft tissue balancing is especially important in patients with a varus coronal plane deformity and may be assessed intraoperatively with a variety of modalities including spacer blocks, laminar spreaders, tensioning devices, and trial components [10].

One study compared 27 knees in 20 patients with preoperative varus deformity 20° or greater to a control group with less than 5° of varus deformity. They found that the varus group had higher variability of results and operative times that were 30 min longer on average, with a knee evaluation score that was not statistically significant difference, and an average postoperative alignment that tended to be in residual varus (3°) [11]. It is important to avoid positioning the tibial component more than 3° varus as this has been demonstrated to increase the likelihood of early failure, usually further to varus caused by medial bone collapse [12].

Management of the PCL (and even the ACL) is a matter of surgeon training, experience, and preference. Proponents of the PCL-sparing philosophy note improved proprioception [13], a bone and soft tissue sparing workflow, and excellent long-term survivorship [14]. Cruciate substitution is cited as a reproducible workflow for the spectrum of ligament loss and is favored by some for its reproducible and consistent femoral rollback [15, 16]. Constrained condylar components offer another element of increased stability. Hinged implants are useful in patients with severe ligamentous insufficiency, or flexion or extension gap mismatch [9].

1.6   Clinical Pearls/Pitfalls

- Consider unicompartmental knee arthroplasty even in patients with severe varus deformity as long as they have an intact ACL, fully correctable deformity, and full thickness lateral cartilage.
- Rotational alignment of TKA femoral component according to AP axis and epicondylar axis is crucial for balancing varus knee, without the need for excessive ligamentous release.

- Tibial component should not be positioned more than 3° varus or else knee is likely to fail further to varus.
- Constrained components or hinged components are reserved for those patients with absent collateral ligaments or excessive flexion gaps.

References

1. Wheeless CR. TKR: fixed varus deformity. In: Wheeless CR, editor. Wheeless' Textbook of orthopaedics. 2013. [cited Nov 15 2014]. Available from: http://www.wheelessonline.com/ortho/tkr_fixed_varus_deformity
2. Virolainen P, Aro HT. High Tibial Osteotomy for the treatment of osteoarthritis of the knee: a review of the literature and a meta-analysis of follow-up studies. Arch Orthop Trauma Surg. 2004;124(4):258–61.
3. Carr A, Keyes G, Miller R, O'Connor J, Goodfellow J. Medial unicompartmental arthroplasty. A survival study of the Oxford meniscal knee. Clin Orthop Relat Res. 1993;295:205–13.
4. Pandit H, Liddle AD, Kendrick BJL, Jenkins C, Price AJ, Gill HS, Dodd CAF, Murray DW. Improved fixation in cementless unicompartmental knee replacement: 5 year results of a randomized controlled trial. J Bone Joint Surg Am. 2013;95:1365–72.
5. Liddle AD, Pandit H, O'Brien S, Doran E, Penny ID, Hooper GJ, Burn PJ, Dodd CAF, Beverland DE, Maxwell AR, Murray DW. Cementless fixation in Oxford unicompartmental knee replacement: a multicentre study of 1000 knees. Bone Joint J. 2013;95-b:181–7.
6. Berend KR, Lombardi Jr AV, Mallory TH, et al. Early failure of minimally invasive unicompartmental knee arthroplasty is associated with obesity. Clin Orthop Relat Res. 2005;440:60.
7. Bolognesi MP, Greiner MA, Attarian DE, Watters TS, Wellman SS, Curtis LH, Berend KR, Setoguchi S. Unicompartmental knee arthroplasty and total knee arthroplasty among medicare beneficiaries, 2000 to 2009. J Bone Joint Surg Am. 2013;95, e174(1–9).
8. Nagamine R, White SE, McCarthy DS, Whiteside LA. Effect of rotational malposition of the femoral component on knee stability kinematics after total knee arthroplasty. J Arthroplasty. 1995;10(3):265–70.

9. Cockarell Jr JR, Guyton JL. Arthroplasty of the knee. In: Canale ST, Beaty JH, editors. Campbell's operative orthopaedics. 11th ed. Philadelphia: Mosby Elsevier; 2008.

10. Mihalko WM, Saleh KJ, Krackow KA, Whiteside LA. Soft-tissue balancing during total knee arthroplasty in the varus knee. J Am Acad Orthop Surg. 2009;17(12):766–74.

11. Teeny SM, Krackow KA, Hungerford DS, Jones M. Primary total knee arthroplasty in patients with severe varus deformity. A comparative study. Clin Orthop Relat Res. 1991;273:19–31.

12. Berend ME, Ritter MA, Meding JB, Faris PM, Keating EM, Redelman R, Faris GW, Davis KE. Tibial component failure mechanisms in total knee arthroplasty. Clin Orthop Relat Res. 2004;428:26–34.

13. Dennis DA, Komistek RD, Colwell Jr CE, Ranawat CS, Scott RD, Thornhill TS, et al. In vivo anteroposterior femorotibial translation of total knee arthroplasty: a multicenter analysis. Clin Orthop Relat Res. 1998;356:47–57.

14. Ritter MA, Davis KE, Farris A, Keating EM, Faris PM. The Surgeon's role in relative success of PCL-retaining and PCL-substituting total knee arthroplasty. HSS J. 2014;10(2):107–15.

15. Dennis DA, Komistek RD, Mahfouz MR, Haas BD, Stiehl JB. Multicenter determination of in vivo kinematics after total knee arthroplasty. Clin Orthop Relat Res. 2003;416:37–57.

16. Stiehl JB, Dennis DA, Komistek RD, Keblish PA. In vivo kinematic comparison of posterior cruciate ligament retention or sacrifice with a mobile bearing total knee arthroplasty. Am J Knee Surg. 2000;13(1):13–8.

Suggested Reading

Total knee arthroplasty. UpToDate. http://www.uptodate.com/

Chapter 2
Complex Primary Total Knee Arthroplasty: Management of Valgus Knee

Jon O. Wright and Ryan M. Nunley

2.1 Case Presentation

2.1.1 History and Physical

A 69-year-old female presented to clinic with the chief complaint of several years of progressively worsening bilateral knee pain, right greater than left. There was no specific incident that started the pain. On the right side, she felt the pain throughout the whole knee, worst on the lateral aspect. She stated the pain was worse with activity, especially with climbing stairs, and relieved by rest; the patient described the pain as sharp with activity but dull/achy at rest.

The patient was initially treated with activity modification, physical therapy, and daily NSAIDs, which sufficiently managed the pain for several years. However, the pain continued to worsen, and the patient subsequently received several intra-articular corticosteroid injections. The first one provided relief for several months, but the last injection only

J.O. Wright, BS • R.M. Nunley, BA, MD (✉)
Department of Orthopedic Surgery, Washington University
School of Medicine, St. Louis, MO, USA
e-mail: nunleyr@wudosis.wustl.edu

© Springer International Publishing Switzerland 2015   13
B.D. Springer and B.M. Curtin (eds.), *Complex Primary
and Revision Total Knee Arthroplasty: A Clinical Casebook*,
DOI 10.1007/978-3-319-18350-3_2

provided relief for approximately 2 weeks, and so she was referred here to discuss possible TKA.

On physical exam, she was tender to palpation mainly on the lateral and anterior aspect of her right knee, with some pain in the left knee as well, but not as severe. Skin was normal with no prior incisions. On the right side, range of motion was 3–110°, and the knee was stable ligamentously. Overall she had 11° of valgus on both knees. She had a mild limp and mild bilateral effusions. Strength was 5/5 in all muscle groups, sensation was intact to light touch in all distributions, and pulses were intact.

Weight-bearing anteroposterior and lateral X-rays and standard patellofemoral X-rays of the knees were obtained and showed bilateral tricompartmental osteoarthritis, with a valgus deformity of 11° on the right side (see Fig. 2.1).

2.1.2   Management

The patient was diagnosed with end-stage osteoarthritis and, having failed conservative therapy, elected to undergo TKA. On the day of surgery, a medial parapatellar approach was used to access the joint. The distal femoral cut was made in 3° of valgus, and rotational alignment of the femoral component was set in reference to the anteroposterior axis and verified with the transepicondylar axis. The tibial cuts were made, and lateral release of the iliotibial band and the posterolateral capsule lateral to the popliteus tendon was performed to achieve appropriate flexion and extension gaps. Components were cemented in place, and the incision was closed. Shortly after the procedure was completed, the peroneal nerve was evaluated and found to be intact.

2.1.3   Outcome

The patient returned to clinic 4 weeks postoperatively. She was doing well with her recovery. X-rays were obtained which showed femoral and tibial components well affixed and in

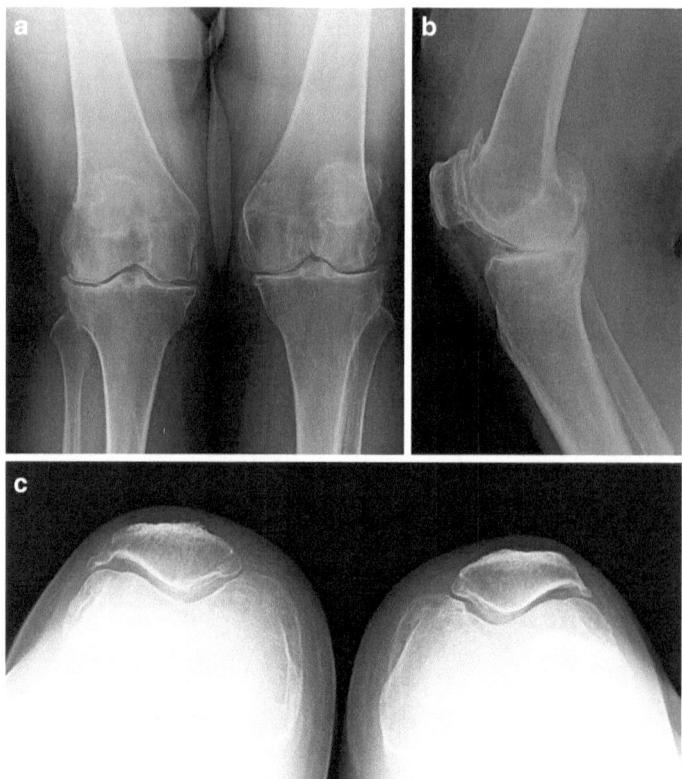

FIG. 2.1. Preoperative X-rays of the knee. View: (**a**) anteroposterior, (**b**) lateral, (**c**) patellofemoral.

near-anatomic alignment (see Fig. 2.2). Standing long-leg anteroposterior films from hip to knee were also obtained and showed the limb corrected to a neutral mechanical alignment (see Fig. 2.3). She was continued on physical therapy to improve strength and range of motion, and she followed up in clinic again 1 year postoperatively, at which point she was still doing well.

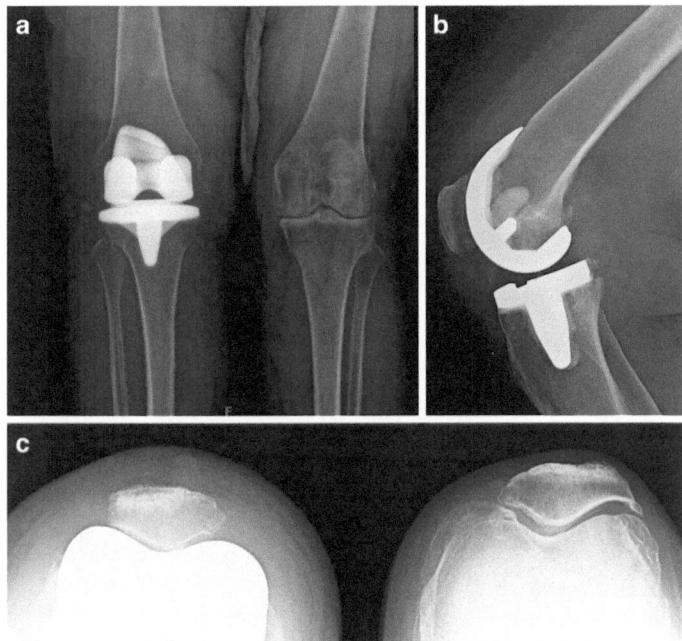

Fig. 2.2. Postoperative X-rays of the knee. Views: (**a**) anteroposterior, (**b**) lateral, (**c**) patellofemoral.

2.2   Literature Review

2.2.1   Introduction

Many surgeons consider total knee arthroplasty (TKA) in the valgus knee to be a more technically difficult procedure than TKA in the varus knee. The increased complexity is partly due to the complex soft tissue releases needed to help create a balanced knee and also partly due to the distal femoral deformity that is commonly encountered. Additionally, clinical decision-making can also be difficult in these cases, as there is no real consensus in the literature as to the best surgical approach and techniques to use, although several different methods have been proposed.

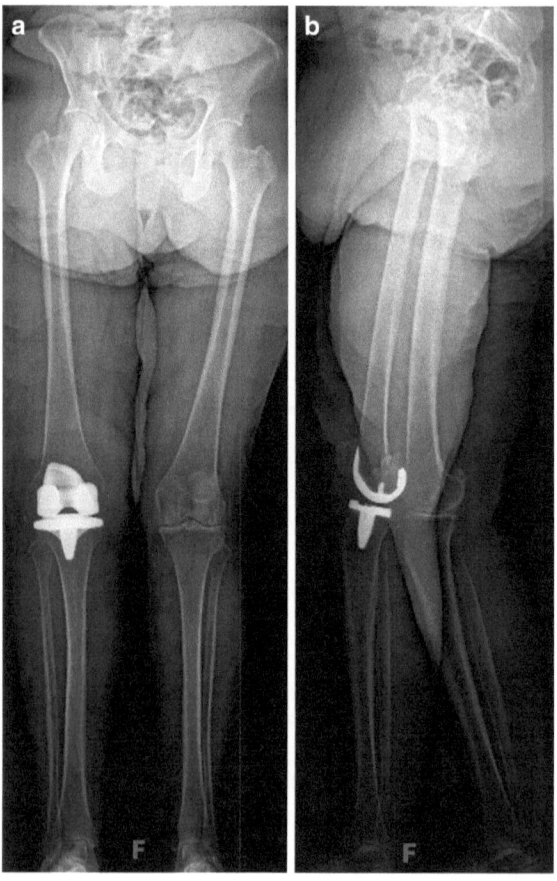

FIG. 2.3. Postoperative standing long-leg X-rays from hip to knee. Views: (**a**) anteroposterior, (**b**) lateral.

Of the various methods proposed in the literature, some of the main areas of discussion include (1) which surgical approach to use, (2) which method to use to properly align the components, (3) how to achieve a final, stable construct through balancing of soft tissues, and (4) selection of an implant with an appropriate degree of constraint. The intent of this chapter is to provide an overview of what has been

TABLE 2.1. Krackow and Ranawat classifications of the valgus knee [1, 2].

Type/variation	Krakow classification	Ranawat classification
I	Valgus deformity secondary to bone loss in the lateral compartment and soft tissue contracture with medial soft tissue still intact	Minimal valgus deformity and minimal soft tissue stretching
II	Like type I except for obvious attenuation of medial capsular ligament complex	Fixed valgus with more substantial deformity (>10 %) and with medial soft tissue stretching
III	Severe deformity with valgus malpositioning of the proximal tibial joint line after overcorrected proximal tibial osteotomy	Severe osseous deformity after a prior osteotomy with an incompetent medial soft tissue sleeve

proposed, helping guide a reader's future study and thereby enabling him or her to make up his or her own mind on each matter.

2.2.2   Classification

Before broaching any of the aforementioned topics, it's worth briefly reviewing the classification systems used for valgus knees (see Table 2.1). The most commonly referenced classification system in North America is probably the Krackow system [1], which categorizes valgus knees based on the integrity of the medial soft tissues and on prior surgeries. A slight variation of this system was described by Ranawat et al. [2] which also takes into consideration the tightness of the lateral soft tissues by assessing whether or not the deformity is fixed or correctable. Other classification systems also exist; however, further discussion of these will not be undertaken here, as most vary only slightly and rely on assessing the same variables: (1) degree of deformity, (2) ability to correct the deformity, (3) medial soft tissue integrity, and (4) history of prior osteotomy.

2.2.3 Technical Aspects Particular to the Valgus Knee

2.2.3.1 Surgical Approach

Either a medial or a lateral approach can be used to access the knee when performing any TKA. The lateral approach is popular in Europe for valgus knees and has several proponents in the US literature [3, 4], although it has not been widely adopted here. The medial approach is more familiar to most surgeons in the United States and is thought to be adequate in all but cases with the most severe deformity.

The fact that it is familiar to most surgeons is one important benefit of choosing the medial approach. Another benefit is that, with this approach, the patella is easy to evert or translate, especially in valgus knees, providing good exposure to the joint without requiring any tibial tuberosity osteotomy. The major disadvantage to this approach is the difficulty of reaching lateral side of the joint in knees with severe valgus deformity, increasing the difficulty of the already somewhat complex lateral release needed to properly balance the knee. Additionally, using this approach risks devascularizing the patella if a too aggressive lateral release is performed and the lateral geniculate arteries are compromised.

The lateral approach has the benefit of direct access to the lateral side of the knee, where the deformity is, without risking the blood supply to the patella, but it is relatively more technically challenging. The main disadvantages to this approach are that (1) a tibial tuberosity osteotomy is often required in order to invert the patella and access the medial side of the knee due to the tuberosity's slightly lateral location on the shaft of the tibia and (2) closure of the retinacular layer becomes problematic after correction of the deformity, necessitating more complex maneuvers such as a Z-cut capsulotomy to develop an adequate tissue layer for final closure.

2.2.3.2   Alignment

When performing any TKA, the main goals of the bony cuts should be to restore the knee joint to a neutral mechanical alignment and to ensure proper rotational alignment of the implants.

The mechanical axis of the leg is defined as the axis from the center of the femoral head to the center of the ankle, which ideally should pass directly through the center of the knee. In a neutrally aligned knee, the difference between the anatomical axis of the femur (defined by a line running down the center of the shaft of the femur) and this mechanical axis is commonly between 5 and 7°, depending upon the length of the patient's femur. In valgus knees, however, the difference between these two axes is increased, and the mechanical axis runs lateral to the center of the knee. In varus knees, it is common for the distal femur to be cut at a valgus angle around 6° to obtain a cut that will be nearly perpendicular to the final mechanical axis of the leg following completion of the surgery. However, in valgus knees, some authors recommend using a smaller angle for the distal femoral cut [2]. This is done to minimally overcorrect for and thereby protect against recurrent valgus deformity, which is a fairly common complication following surgery in these patients.

Once the distal femoral cut has been made to restore a neutral mechanical axis, the next cuts to be made on the femur set the rotational alignment for the implant, which affects both the varus-valgus stability during flexion and determines the position of the patellar groove. Several different axes have been proposed which can be used in reference to attain the proper alignment (see Fig. 2.4).

One of the most commonly used alignment techniques in TKA is to align the components in slight external rotation to the posterior femoral condylar axis, an axis defined by a line connecting the posterior aspects of the femoral condyles. Using this axis gives consistent results in most varus knees. However, this method should be avoided in the valgus knee, as wear and hypoplasia on the lateral femoral condyle can

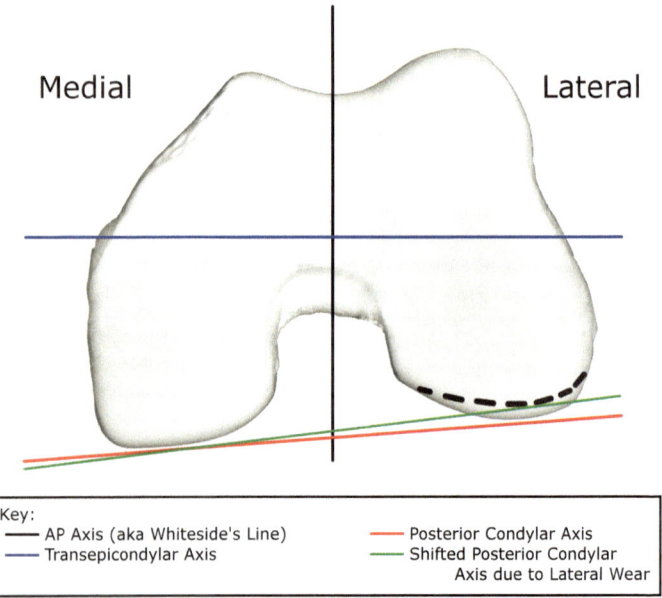

Key:
— AP Axis (aka Whiteside's Line)   — Posterior Condylar Axis
— Transepicondylar Axis   — Shifted Posterior Condylar
                                        Axis due to Lateral Wear

FIG. 2.4. Femoral axes that can be used as a reference for rotational alignment of femoral cuts.

result in altered osseous anatomy and hence an inappropriate reference axis (see Fig. 2.4). Using this method therefore may lead to inappropriate internal rotation of the femoral component and subsequent medial displacement of the patellar groove, resulting in an increased Q angle and potential patellar maltracking.

Two alternate alignment axes, the transepicondylar axis and the anteroposterior axis of the femur (AP axis), have been proposed to avoid this problem. Using cadaveric studies, Berger et al. showed that transepicondylar axis, defined by a line through the lateral epicondylar prominence and the medial sulcus of the medial epicondyle, provides a reliable axis for alignment [5]. However, intraoperatively determining this axis can be rather difficult. Another method to attain proper alignment in the valgus knee was proposed by Arima et al. [6, 7]. They recommended using the anteroposterior axis of the femur (otherwise known as the Whiteside line), defined by a line through the deepest part of the patellar groove anteriorly and the center of the intercondylar notch posteriorly. Their group showed that using this new axis for rotational alignment in patients with valgus knees gave superior clinical results when compared to using the posterior condylar axis, with fewer patients needing tibial tubercle transfers intraoperatively and fewer patients experiencing patellar instability in the years following surgery.

The tibial cuts can usually be approached the same way in the valgus knee as in the varus knee. The transverse cut is made perpendicular to the anatomic axis of the tibia, which is coincident with the ideal mechanical axis of the leg unless there is preexisting tibial deformity. The tibial component is usually placed to have the center of the tibial component in line with the junction of the medial and middle 1/3 of the tibial tubercle. Excessive internal or external rotation will affect the final Q angle and may lead to patellar maltracking and soft tissue irritation postoperatively.

On a final note, release of the tight lateral retinaculum is often needed to obtain neutral patella tracking. As mentioned earlier, care should be taken while doing so if a medial approach has been utilized to avoid sacrificing the lateral geniculate arteries and risk devascularizing the patella.

2.2.3.3   Gap Balancing and Component Selection

Probably the most debated topic regarding TKA in the valgus knee concerns the best way to ensure a final stable construct through means of soft tissue balancing and/or use of constrained components. Most commonly, authors recommend some type of lateral soft tissue release be used in conjunction with either a cruciate retaining or posterior stabilized implant [1]. However, as the degree of deformity increases and medial soft tissue laxity is encountered, the best way to proceed becomes less clear. Authors vary on their approach in these cases, with some recommending various techniques to tighten medial structures, others recommending wider

TABLE 2.2. Whiteside algorithm of lateral soft tissue release for gap balancing [9].

Gap tight laterally in flexion only	Gap tight laterally in extension only	Gap tight laterally in both flexion and extension
1. Release the LCL 2. If the lateral tightness is associated with internal rotational contracture, release the popliteus tendon	1. Release the IT band 2. If still too tight, release the posterolateral capsule	1. Balance first as if tight in flexion only 2. If tightness persists in extension, release the IT band first and then the posterolateral capsule as needed

tibial implants to fill the resultant gap, and finally others who recommend using more constrained implants and avoiding addressing the medial soft tissue laxity.

When proceeding with a lateral soft tissue release, the structures most often released include the iliotibial (IT) band, the posterolateral capsule, the popliteus tendon, the lateral head of the gastrocnemius, and the lateral collateral ligament. However, the recommended order of their release varies by author. Lombardi et al. recommended a simple sequential approach to the release, starting with the IT band and then proceeding sequentially with the posterolateral capsule, popliteus tendon, and then finally the LCL, assessing the gaps and stability of the knee after each successive release until adequate balancing is achieved [8]. Whiteside proposed a more complex algorithm, taking into consideration whether the gap was tight in either flexion, extension, or both [9]. His proposed algorithm can be seen in Table 2.2. Multiple other authors have also offered their own slightly varying recommendations on this topic. Adding to the difficulty of choosing a method to follow, not only does one have to choose which structures and in which order to perform the release, the technique of how to perform the release is also debated. While some authors propose simple transection of the structures, others propose using a so-called "pie-crusting" technique, wherein the surgeon makes multiple transverse stab incisions in the posterolateral tissues being released, as a way to facilitate the required release of tension without completely transecting the structures [10]. Several variations using this "pie-crusting" technique exist in the literature, once again differing by the sequence of structures to be addressed. Clinical outcome studies have been reported on all of these above-mentioned techniques and on multiple others as well, and most have been shown to produce reasonable outcomes.

In more complicated cases where both lateral contraction and medial laxity are combined, the surgeon has an even more difficult decision to make. Some authors propose that cases of minimal medial laxity can be treated simply by increasing the thickness of the tibial insert. However, severe valgus deformity may result in too large of a gap to feasibly fill with the tibial insert if lateral release is simply carried out to match the medial laxity. That leaves the surgeon with two different options to attain the needed stability of the final construct, either attempting to tighten the lax medial soft tissues or opting to use a more constrained implant.

Several authors have addressed the first method, recommending various procedures to tighten the insufficient MCL. They report satisfactory results while still using less-constrained implants [1], thus better preserving the natural mechanics of the knee. However, these methods can be technically challenging and add time to the operation, both of which increase the risk to the patient. Other authors argue against addressing the medial structures at all, but rather recommend the second method, using a more constrained prostheses to attain a stable construct. In a more extreme example of this, Easley et al. showed that in an elderly population, using a more constrained implant, the constrained condylar knee, without addressing medial tissue laxity nor even performing any lateral soft tissue release, gave reasonable results while avoiding longer surgeries and the possible complications associated with both lateral release and medial tightening [11].

2.2.4   Complications in the Valgus Knee

Certain complications have been shown to be more common in patients with valgus knees undergoing TKA when compared to TKA patients with varus knees, several of which deserve specific mention:

- Patellar osteonecrosis—As mentioned above, this is particularly a problem when extensive lateral release is done in conjunction with a medial surgical approach. Those electing this surgical approach should be aware of this potential complication and ensure that they do not transect the lateral geniculate arteries during their release in order to preserve the blood supply to the patella.
- Patellar tracking problems—The higher incidence of this in patients with valgus knees is possibly due to the difficulty of attaining correct rotational alignment of the implants. To avoid this, the posterior condylar axis should not be used as a reference, and the surgeon should be proficient at using either the transepicondylar axis or the AP axis to correctly align the femoral prosthesis.
- Peroneal nerve palsy—In most cases, this is thought to be due to release and subsequent lengthening of the lateral soft tissue, resulting in excessive traction to the nerve [12]. If palsy is discovered, the knee should be immediately placed in flexion to decrease traction on the nerve and any constrictive dressings should be removed. Of note, the peroneal nerve is also particularly at risk if the "pie-crusting" technique is used on the posterolateral capsule, so the surgeon should be cognizant of this risk intraoperatively and take appropriate care.

2.3   Clinical Pearls/Pitfalls

- Good results can be achieved through various different methods when performing TKA in the valgus knee. A surgeon should be aware of the various techniques that have been proposed and use them according to his or her best clinical judgment.

- Referencing the posterior condylar axis should be avoided in valgus knees, as excessive lateral femoral condylar wear or lateral femoral condyle hypoplasia can lead to excessive internal rotation of the implant if this axis is used.
- Although the absolute risk is small, patients with valgus knees are particularly at risk for peroneal nerve palsy following TKA. Function of the nerve should be assessed as soon as possible postoperatively, and some people would advocate avoiding long-acting spinal anesthesia in these patients to allow for early assessment of nerve function in the recovery room.

References

1. Krackow KA, Jones MM, Teeny SM, Hungerford DS. Primary total knee arthroplasty in patients with fixed valgus deformity. Clin Orthop Relat Res. 1991;273(273):9–18.
2. Ranawat AS, Ranawat CS, Elkus M, Rasquinha VJ, Rossi R, Babhulkar S. Total knee arthroplasty for severe valgus deformity. J Bone Joint Surg Am. 2005;87 Suppl 1(Pt 2):271–84.
3. Apostolopoulos AP, Nikolopoulos DD, Polyzois I, Nakos A, Liarokapis S, Stefanakis G, et al. Total knee arthroplasty in severe valgus deformity: interest of combining a lateral approach with a tibial tubercle osteotomy. Orthop Traumatol Surg Res. 2010;96(7):777–84.
4. Keblish PA. The lateral approach to the valgus knee. Surgical technique and analysis of 53 cases with over two-year follow-up evaluation. Clin Orthop Relat Res. 1991;271:52–62.
5. Berger RA, Rubash HE, Seel MJ, Thompson WH, Crossett LS. Determining the rotational alignment of the femoral component in total knee arthroplasty using the epicondylar axis. Clin Orthop Relat Res. 1993;286:40–7.
6. Arima J, Whiteside LA, McCarthy DS, White SE. Femoral rotational alignment, based on the anteroposterior axis, in total knee arthroplasty in a valgus knee. A technical note. J Bone Joint Surg Am. 1995;77(9):1331–4.
7. Whiteside LA, Arima J. The anteroposterior axis for femoral rotational alignment in valgus total knee arthroplasty. Clin Orthop Relat Res. 1995;321:168–72.

8. Lombardi AV, Dodds KL, Berend KR, Mallory TH, Adams JB. An algorithmic approach to total knee arthroplasty in the valgus knee. J Bone Joint Surg Am. 2004;86-A(Suppl):62–71.
9. Whiteside LA. Selective ligament release in total knee arthroplasty of the knee in valgus. Clin Orthop Relat Res. 1999;367: 130–40.
10. Elkus M, Ranawat CS, Rasquinha VJ, Babhulkar S, Rossi R, Ranawat AS. Total knee arthroplasty for severe valgus deformity. Five to fourteen-year follow-up. J Bone Joint Surg Am. 2004;86-A(12):2671–6.
11. Easley ME, Insall JN, Scuderi GR, Bullek DD. Primary constrained condylar knee arthroplasty for the arthritic valgus knee. Clin Orthop Relat Res. 2000;380(380):58–64.
12. Favorito PJ, Mihalko WM, Krackow KA. Total knee arthroplasty in the valgus knee. J Am Acad Orthop Surg. 2002;10(1):16–24.

Chapter 3
Complex Primary Total Knee Arthroplasty: Management of Flexion Contracture

Gregory G. Polkowski

3.1 Case Presentation

The patient is a 66-year-old male veteran with a 15-year history of progressive right knee pain. As a serviceman, he sustained periodic "knee sprains" which were managed non-surgically with conservative treatment. In his 50s he underwent a total of three knee arthroscopy procedures for meniscal debridement and chondroplasty which provided him with an improvement in symptoms. Since developing osteoarthritis, he has been treated with physical therapy and multiple intra-articular corticosteroid injections, which of recent have failed to provide substantial pain relief. He presents with increasing pain and diminished function.

On physical examination, the patient stands 5 ft 11 in. tall weighing 200 lb and walks with a limp reflective of his fairly stiff right knee. He lacks 20° of full extension actively and passively (Fig. 3.1) and flexes his knee to 95° only. He has substantial coronal plane varus deformity that is fixed in nature. His extensor mechanism function and quadriceps strength are normal, as is the remainder of his physical examination.

G.G. Polkowski, MD, MSc (✉)
Department of Orthopedic Surgery, Vanderbilt University Medical
Center, Nashville, TN, USA
e-mail: gregory.polkowski@vanderbilt.edu

© Springer International Publishing Switzerland 2015   29
B.D. Springer and B.M. Curtin (eds.), *Complex Primary
and Revision Total Knee Arthroplasty: A Clinical Casebook*,
DOI 10.1007/978-3-319-18350-3_3

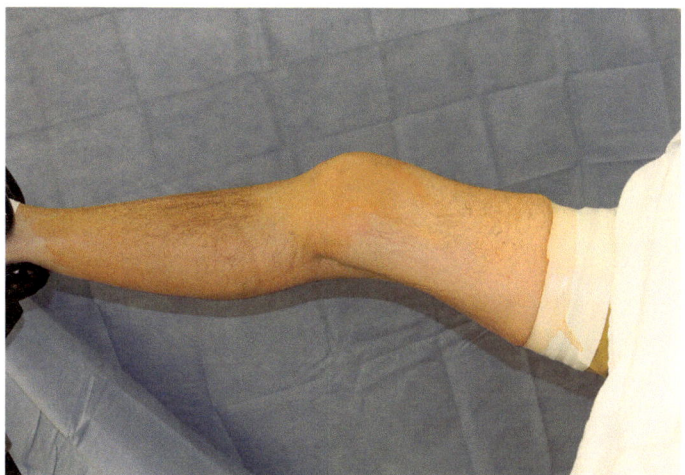

FIG. 3.1. Lateral picture of the patient's right knee after surgical prep depicting 20° flexion contracture.

Weight-bearing AP, lateral, and sunrise radiographs of the patient's right knee showed advanced joint space narrowing, subchondral sclerosis, and abundant osteophyte formation, all consistent with a diagnosis of osteoarthritis (Fig. 3.2). As the patient had previously undergone exhaustive nonsurgical treatment and was substantially limited by his pain and stiffness, he was interested in pursuing total knee arthroplasty surgery.

3.2   Diagnosis/Assessment

The patient's history, physical and radiographic findings are consistent with the diagnosis of advanced osteoarthritis with a fixed varus deformity and flexion contracture. While the presence of coronal plane deformity is common in most knees requiring total knee arthroplasty, the presence of substantial (greater than 15°) flexion contractures is not as common and deserves special consideration for operative planning. Such flexion contractures need to be addressed during TKA

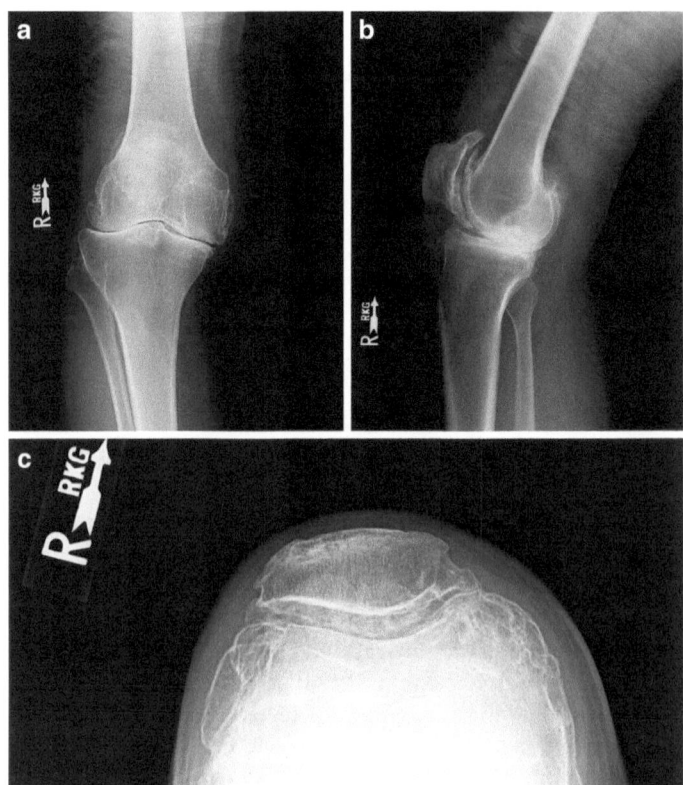

FIG. 3.2. Preoperative standing AP, lateral, and sunrise views. (a) Standing AP radiograph showing joint space obliteration, peripheral osteophytosis, and medial tibial bone loss. (b) Lateral radiograph showing substantial patellar and posterior femoral osteophyte formation, along with posterior translation of the femur on the tibia. (c) Sunrise radiographs showing patellofemoral osteoarthritis with severe peripheral patellar osteophytosis, but appropriate patellar tracking.

surgery to ensure optimal postoperative range of motion, normal gait mechanics, and good patient satisfaction.

In general, flexion contractures during TKA surgery can be managed by utilizing one or a combination of the following techniques: (1) Coronal plane balancing with collateral ligament releases as needed; (2) Complete resection of posterior osteophytes and subsequent posterior capsular releasing as needed; (3) Resection of additional distal femoral bone; and (4) Hamstring muscle tenotomy. While many of these techniques are used in combination with one another, each case must be taken on an individual basis, as subtle radiographic and physical examination findings can help direct the surgeon through the ideal sequence of releases and bone resection that result and a well-balanced fully extended knee.

3.3   Management

An initial medial parapatellar arthrotomy was performed for exposure, with severe osteoarthritic findings being confirmed upon inspection of the joint (Fig. 3.3). The extensive patellar osteophytes were resected to help enhance patellar mobilization, and an extramedullary guide was used to resect approximately 10 mm of tibial bone referencing the more intact lateral tibial plateau (Fig. 3.4). A distal femoral resection of 10 mm was performed (standard resection is 8 mm) (Fig. 3.5),

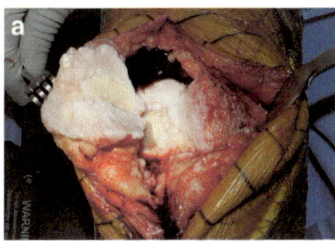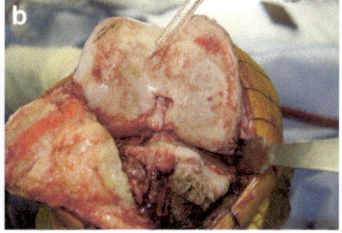

Fig. 3.3. Intraoperative photos. (**a**) Intraoperative photo showing hyper-osteophytic knee with extensive peripatellar, tibial, and femoral osteophytes. (**b**) After resection of patellar osteophytes the patella was everted, the knee flexed, and the remainder of the joint exposed. Posterior medial tibial bone loss is evident and consistent with the patient's preoperative clinical findings of fixed varus deformity.

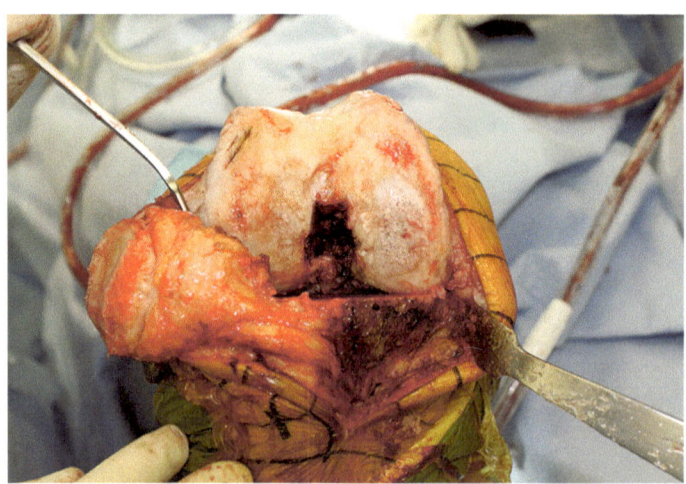

Fig. 3.4. Intraoperative photograph after tibial resection of 10 mm referencing the intact lateral plateau using an extramedullary tibial guide.

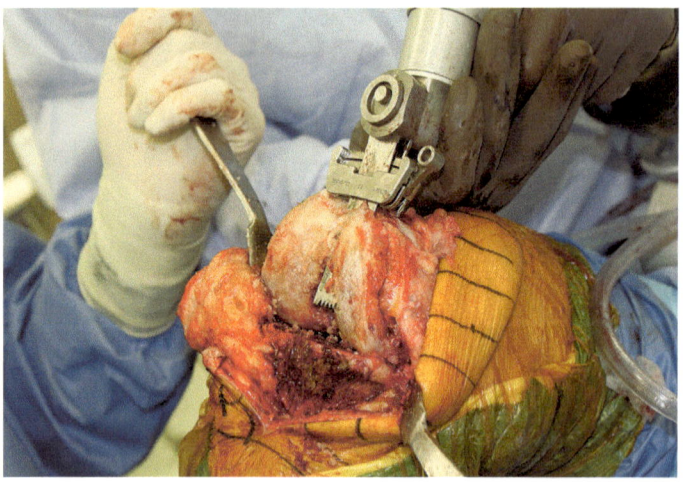

Fig. 3.5. Intraoperative photograph showing initial distal femoral resection of 10 mm, which is 2 mm greater than the thickness of implant on distal femur (8 mm).

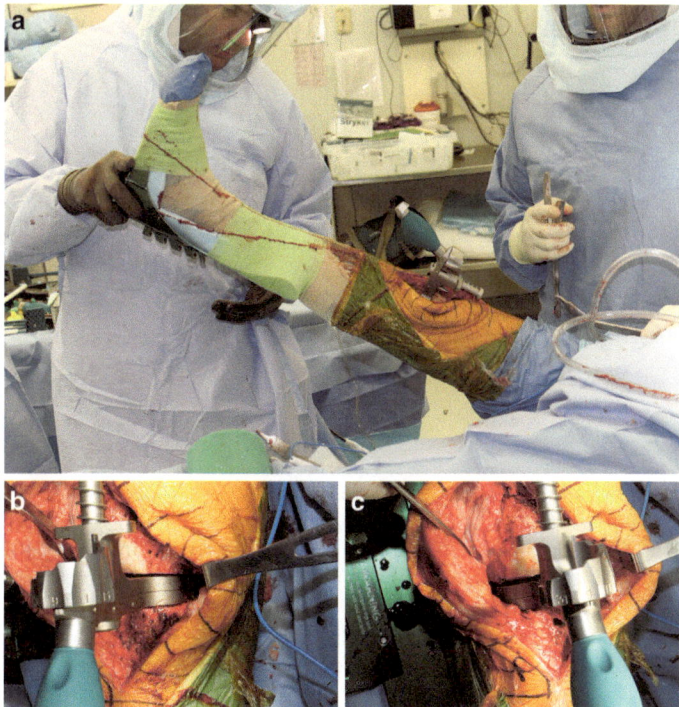

Fig. 3.6. Intraoperative assessment of extension space with spacer block. (**a**) Full extension was achieved with the minimal thickness spacer block, which represents the composite thickness of the implants and the smallest 9 mm polyethylene insert. (**b**) In extension, the knee was tight medially with no gapping when a valgus force was applied. (**c**) The lateral compartment, however, was loose and would eventually require a thicker polyethylene to accommodate the laxity in this location.

and the knee balance was assessed in full extension (Fig. 3.6a). A 9 mm equivalent spacer block (minimal composite implant/polyethylene thickness) was inserted which revealed tight medial space (Fig. 3.6b), and relative lateral laxity that would accommodate a 13 mm equivalent polyethylene (Fig. 3.6c).

The remainder of the femoral cuts were performed, with the external rotation of the femoral component being set in

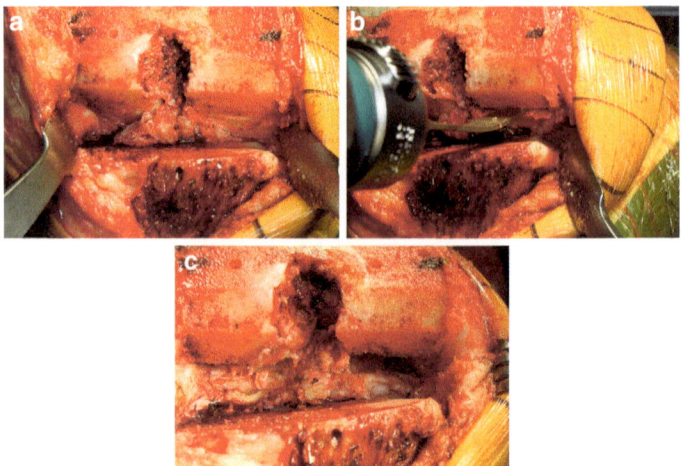

FIG. 3.7. Posterior joint space after femoral cutting block removed. (**a**) The flexion space is assessed with the posterior femur elevated. Extensive posterior osteophytes are seen along the cut surfaces of both posterior femoral condyles. (**b**) A curved osteotome was used to resect the osteophytes from the posterior condyles of the femur. (**c**) Posterior condyles and flexion space after resection of osteophytes. The persistent coronal plane imbalance is evident with the medial side being tighter than the lateral.

alignment with the epicondylar axis, which in this case was approximately 4° externally rotated from the posterior condylar axis. Inspection of the posterior joint space revealed extensive posterior osteophyte formation (Fig. 3.7a). A curved osteotome was used to resect the posterior osteophytes along with some additional posterior condylar bone (Fig. 3.7b, c). A posterior medial release of the tibial semimembranosus tendon insertion was also performed, along with a carefully titrated pie crusting of the superficial medial collateral ligament with an 18-gauge needle to help balance the knee in the coronal plane (Fig. 3.8). With the coronal plane balance accomplished, the flexion and extension spaces were again checked and trial components inserted. A 13 mm polyethylene insert gave appropriate soft tissue tension in flexion, but the knee would not fully extend (Fig. 3.9), so a posterior

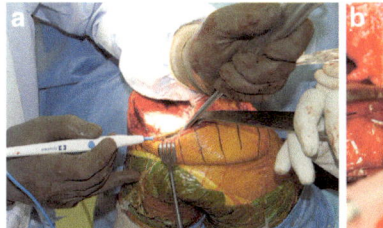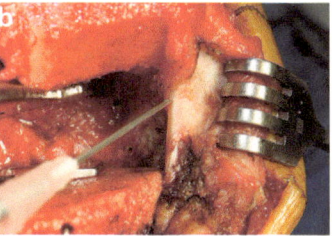

FIG. 3.8. Medial sided releases to help correct coronal plane imbalance. (**a**) A posterior medial release along the tibial joint line including semimembranosus insertion along the posterior medial aspect of the tibia was performed with electrocautery and Cobb elevator. (**b**) After posterior medial release, the knee remained tight medially, and so a carefully titrated release of portions of the superficial medial collateral ligament was performed with an 18-gauge needle, a process which achieved excellent coronal plane balance.

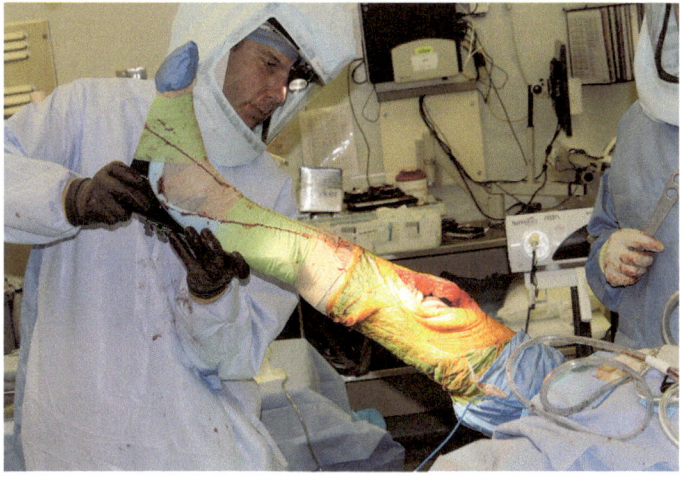

FIG. 3.9. Lateral picture with trial implants and a 13 mm polyethylene liner in place. The knee would not fully extend, but the 13 mm liner gave appropriate soft tissue tension in flexion.

capsular release was performed with electrocautery and a Cobb elevator (Fig. 3.10). The trial implants were inserted again, and the knee would fully extend with a 13 mm

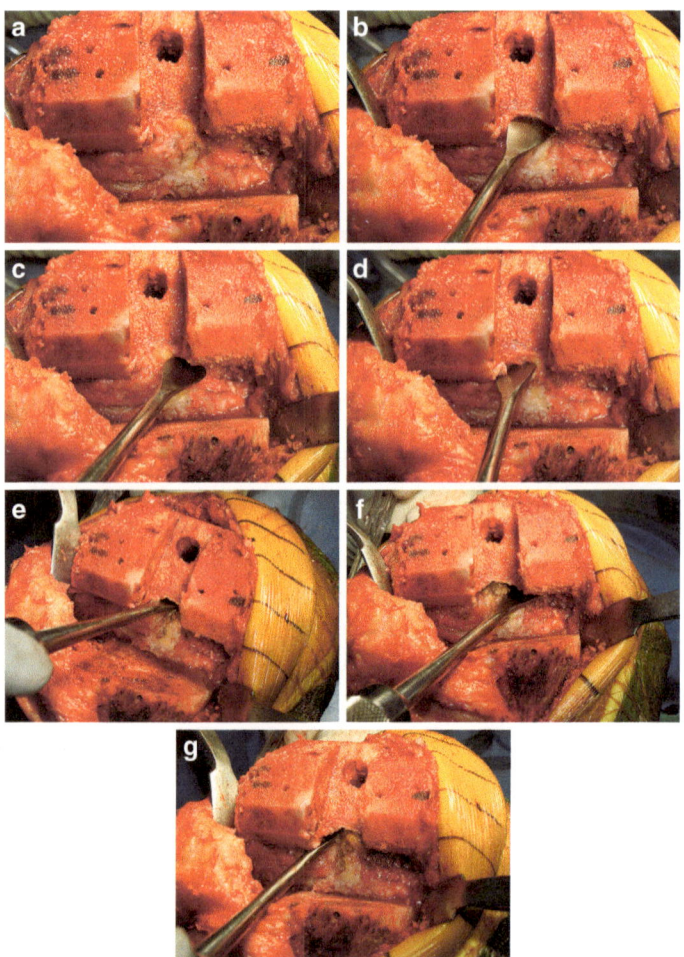

FIG. 3.10. Posterior capsule release. (**a**) View of flexion space after coronal plane balancing showing rectangular flexion gap and intact posterior capsule. (**b–d**) Cobb elevator showing locations for central, medial, and lateral portions of posterior capsular releases (respectively) using electrocautery, and trajectory of Cobb elevator releasing along posterior femur. (**e–g**) Cobb elevator *after* posterior capsular release showing extent and trajectory of release in the central, medial, and lateral portions of the posterior capsule, respectively.

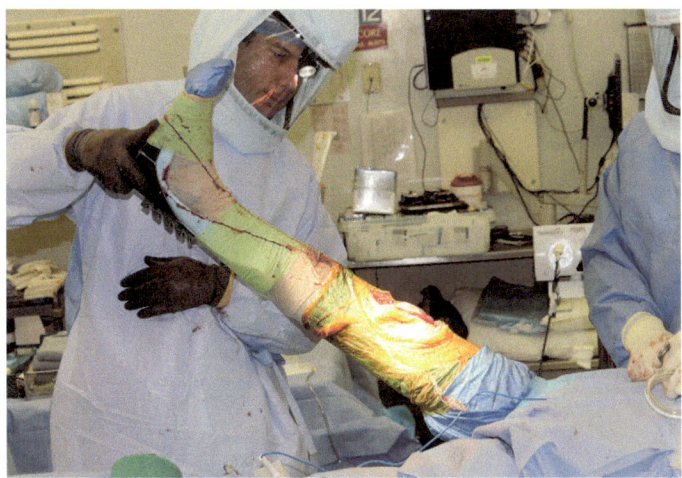

FIG. 3.11. After posterior capsule release, and reinsertion of trial components with 13 mm polyethylene, the knee remained well balanced in flexion, and would now fully extend with gravity alone.

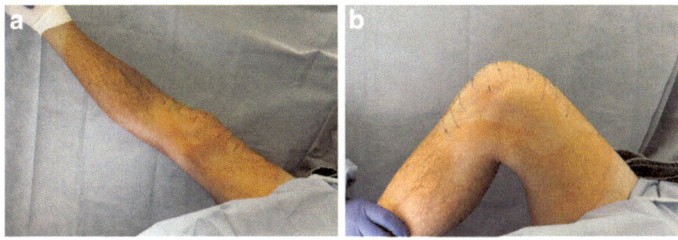

FIG. 3.12. Lateral view of knee after closure. (**a**) Full extension was achieved with gravity alone, the considerable improvement compared with preoperative state (Fig. 3.1). (**b**) Removal of posterior osteophytes and patellofemoral osteophytes allowed for substantial improvement in knee flexion compared with preoperative motion of only 90°.

polyethylene insert (Fig. 3.11). The implants were cemented into place, and the wound was closed in the usual fashion. Prior to application of dressing, the knee would fully extend after wound closure and easily flex past 120° (Fig. 3.12).

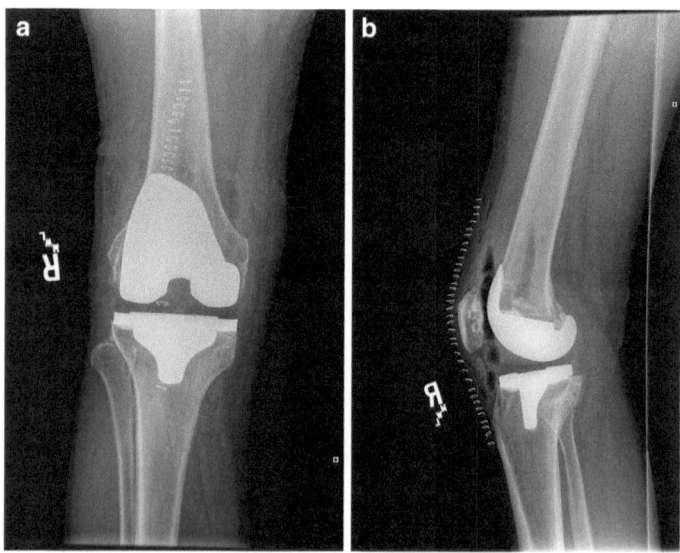

Fig. 3.13. Postoperative radiographs. (**a**) AP radiograph of knee shows normal postoperative changes with neutral mechanical alignment on this limited view. (**b**) Lateral radiograph shows appropriate tibial and femoral component alignment with removal of all posterior knee osteophytes.

Postoperative radiographs show appropriate alignment of total knee components (Fig. 3.13).

In summary, for the patient presented in this case with a 20° flexion contracture, fixed varus deformity, and substantial posterior osteophytes, the following sequence of actions was taken to help insure good knee balance: (1) Resection of an additional 2 mm of distal femoral bone with initial distal femur cut; (2) Resection of posterior femoral osteophytes; (3) Coronal plane balancing with extensive posterior medial release including semimembranosus insertion and slight pie crusting of superficial MCL with an 18-gauge needle; and (4) Posterior capsular release with electrocautery and a Cobb elevator.

3.4 Outcome

This 66-year-old gentleman with preoperative flexion contracture and a fixed varus deformity presented in this case recovered uneventfully, and was able to maintain full extension throughout his recovery period. At 4 months postoperative, his range of motion was from 0 to 125° flexion, and he was able to ambulate without a limp.

3.5 Literature Review

There is a relative paucity of data in the orthopedic literature on the clinical outcome of patients with substantial preoperative flexion contractures prior to TKA, but a few case series do exist. Berend and colleagues reported on 52 knees with preoperative flexion contractures greater than 20° that were managed successfully with less than 10° residual flexion contracture at a mean follow-up of 37 months [1]. In 60 % of these cases, a cruciate retaining prosthesis was used, a PS design was used in 30%, and constrained type implants or rotating hinge prostheses used in the remaining 14 %. Whiteside and Mihalko also reported a large case series of 542 knees with preoperative contractures greater than 10°. The authors reported success in 95 % of the cases and emphasized coronal plane ligament balancing and osteophyte removal, rather than posterior capsular releasing and additional distal femoral bone resection to help manage flexion contractures, practices that were only required in 3 % and 2 % of the cases, respectively [2]. Bellemans and colleagues also described their experience with both moderate (15–30° preoperative contracture) and severe (greater than 30°) contractures using a process similar to that described in the case above, with coronal plane balancing and an initial 2 mm additional distal femur resection emphasized first, followed by posterior capsular releasing, and only then additional distal femur resection and hamstring tenotomy [3]. At 2 years, all patients had less than 10° persistent contracture.

3.6   Clinical Pearls/Pitfalls

- The key to the management of the total knee with a preoperative flexion contracture is not to initially resect too much distal femoral bone without first evaluating the posterior osteophytes/capsule and the steps that may be necessary to balance the knee in the coronal plane.
- Excessive distal femoral resection (>4 mm beyond the minimum for a given implant system) is not recommended, as raising the joint line to that extent affects collateral ligament balance and can lead to mid-flexion instability.
- Additionally, over-resection of the distal femur too soon in the total knee process may lead to extension laxity compared with flexion, if the steps taken for coronal plane balancing and posterior osteophyte resection lead to a greater degree of knee extension than the surgeon anticipates. As such, the author recommends an additional 2 mm distal femoral resection with the initial distal femoral cut, followed by osteophyte resection and coronal plane balancing, then posterior capsular releasing prior to additional distal femoral resection.
- In cases of severe contracture, in addition to these techniques, hamstring tenotomy may be necessary in rare circumstances.

References

1. Berend KR, Lombardi Jr AV, Adams JB. Total knee arthroplasty in patients with greater than 20 degrees flexion contracture. Clin Orthop Relat Res. 2006;452:83–7.
2. Whiteside LA, Mihalko WM. Surgical procedure for flexion contracture and recurvatum in total knee arthroplasty. Clin Orthop Relat Res. 2002;404:189–95.
3. Bellemans J, Vandenneucker H, Victor J, Vanlauwe J. Flexion contracture in total knee arthroplasty. Clin Orthop Relat Res. 2006;452:78–82.

Chapter 4
Complex Primary Total Knee Arthroplasty: Management of Previous Hardware (Posttraumatic OA)

Juan C. Suarez and Raúl G. Gösthe

4.1 Case Presentation

A 50-year-old male presented with a several year history of progressive left knee pain. Past history is significant for a closed tibia fracture in 2010 from a motor vehicle accident requiring open reduction and internal fixation. He denied any perioperative complications such as prolonged wound drainage or antibiotic treatment. Physical examination revealed a midline scar over the knee extending into the proximal tibia with a passively correctable varus knee deformity. His knee range of motion was 0–110°. Radiographic evaluation showed advanced posttraumatic tricompartmental degenerative joint disease with a long laterally based tibial plate with multiple distal broken screws (see Fig. 4.1). Serologic evaluation showed an erythrocyte sedimentation

J.C. Suarez, MD (✉)
Orthopedic and Rheumatologic Institute, Cleveland Clinic Florida, Weston, FL, USA
e-mail: suarezj@ccf.org

R.G. Gösthe, MD
Orthopedic Surgery, Jackson Memorial Hospital/University of Miami, Miami, FL, USA

© Springer International Publishing Switzerland 2015   43
B.D. Springer and B.M. Curtin (eds.), *Complex Primary and Revision Total Knee Arthroplasty: A Clinical Casebook*, DOI 10.1007/978-3-319-18350-3_4

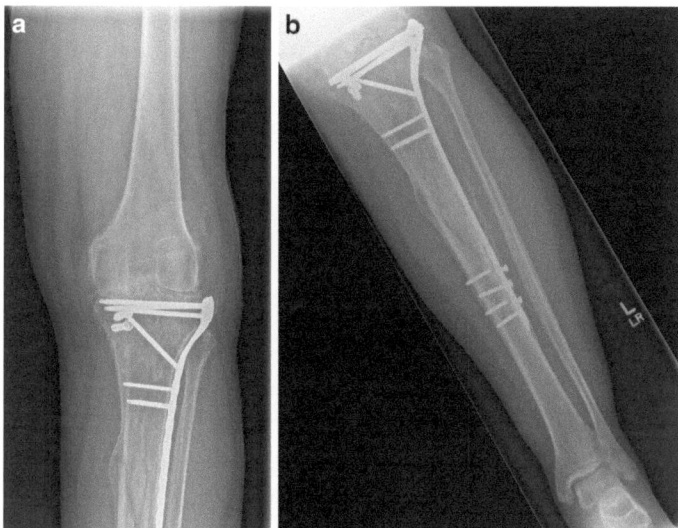

Fig. 4.1. (**a** and **b**) AP radiographs reveal posttraumatic arthritis with retained lateral tibia locking plate with broken distal cortical screws.

rate (ESR) of 72 mm/h and C-reactive protein (CRP) of 20.4 mg/L. Knee aspiration revealed a white blood cell count of 86 cells/μL with 11 % neutrophils and negative cultures.

4.1.1   Diagnosis

The patient presented with severe posttraumatic arthritis and retained hardware. Despite a benign history and knee aspiration, the serologic evaluation was concerning for occult infection. The knee aspiration, although negative, may be unreliable due to the extra-articular nature of the hardware. Consideration was made to perform a staged approach to the reconstruction with removal of hardware and antibiotic treatment prior to definite reconstruction in anticipation of periprosthetic infection.

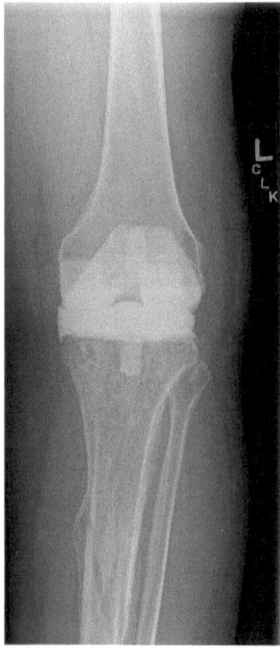

Fig. 4.2. Postoperative AP radiograph with complete hardware removal and resection arthroplasty with articulating antibiotic cement spacer.

4.1.2   Management

The patient underwent a resection arthroplasty and complete removal of the hardware with placement of an articulating antibiotic cement spacer (see Fig. 4.2). Intraoperative frozen sections of the synovial tissue and perihardware tissue revealed significant acute inflammation with microabscesses consistent with infection. A universal screw removal set and high-speed metal-cutting burrs were required for complete hardware removal. Intraoperative cultures were negative and the patient received 6 weeks of broad-spectrum intravenous antibiotics, after which his serologic markers normalized. Final reconstruction was performed thereafter using stemmed implants to bypass stress risers (see Fig. 4.3).

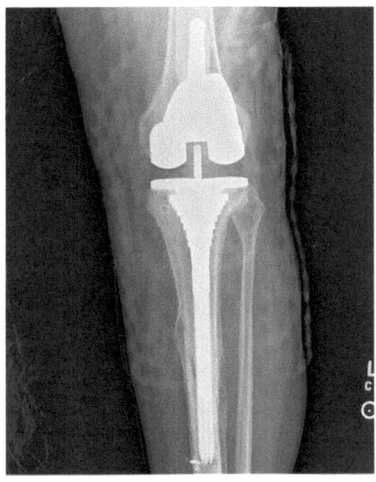

Fɪɢ. 4.3. Postoperative AP radiograph after arthroplasty reconstruction with long-stem components.

4.2   Literature Review

4.2.1   Preoperative Considerations

Complete evaluation of the posttraumatic knee requires a through history of the events surrounding the prior injury, surgery, and any perioperative complications. The physical examination includes evaluation of prior incisions and baseline range of motion, ligamentous stability, and skeletal deformity. Radiographic evaluation consists of a standard weight-bearing knee series as well as full-length femur and tibia views, if necessary, to visualize hardware completely as well as any extra-articular deformities.

4.2.2   Periprosthetic Infection

Periprosthetic joint infection remains a feared complication with significant negative implications for the patient and surgeon alike. Although the typical incidence of periprosthetic infection is quoted as <2 % in the primary setting, this number can exceed 12 % in high risk groups [2]. Suzuki et al. reported that previous open reduction with internal fixation and retained internal fixation hardware was found to be an independent risk factor to the development of periprosthetic joint infections. In contrast to this study, however, Klatte et al. found no increased risk of periprosthetic joint infection in patients with pre-existing osteosynthesis hardware at 5.4 years follow-up of 115 patients they studied [3]. Regardless, the debilitating consequences of periprosthetic joint infections require one to maintain a high index of suspicion of occult infection in the presence of previous internal fixation. History of open fractures, persistent wound drainage, and previous antibiotic treatment following ORIF should raise concerns of chronic infection. Routine serologic evaluation with a complete blood count, erythrocyte sedimentation rate, and C-reactive protein should be obtained. Elevated values and/or high clinical suspicion should prompt a knee aspiration. It is important to recognize, however, that a negative aspiration does not eliminate the possibility of an infection of in situ hardware, as the hardware may be extra-articular. Additional nuclear medicine imaging, such as a white blood cell labeled scan, can be of value if the diagnosis is in question. A positive infection workup, or high clinical suspicion, should trigger a two-stage approach with complete hardware removal, thorough debridement, and tailored intravenous antibiotic treatment. The arthroplasty procedure should be delayed until infection has been ruled out or resolved.

4.3   Surgical Planning

4.3.1   Hardware Management

As a general rule, we recommend removing symptomatic hardware or that which interferes with the preparation for, or implantation of, the total knee arthroplasty. Complete removal is often unnecessary in many instances. In general, this can be accomplished in a single-stage operation. This allows for less surgical morbidity, decreased soft tissue dissection, and prevents creation of unnecessary stress risers. When multiple incisions are anticipated for hardware removal, a staged approach should be entertained to allow the soft tissues to heal prior to the arthroplasty procedure. In order to facilitate hardware removal, complete understanding of implants in place, their location, and any post-traumatic deformities should be part of the surgical planning. To do so, full-length radiographic evaluation of the tibia and femur is often required. In addition, previous operative reports can clarify what specific implants are in place, so that appropriate removal sets can be requested. Often, however, the hardware is unidentified or damaged and one must therefore be equipped with comprehensive hardware extraction sets. A universal screw removal set and high-speed cutting burrs (e.g., Midas Rex) can facilitate hardware extraction and should be available (see Fig. 4.1b). The presence of hardware does not simply provide an obstacle in its removal, but also in implant selection for the arthroplasty.

4.3.2   Implant Selection

Part of the surgical planning is anticipating the need for revision implants. As aforementioned, hardware removal frequently creates stress risers. One must anticipate bone loss associated with prior fracture that may require use of either metallic or bone augments. In such settings, stem augmentation is recommended to support deficient bone and bypass the stress risers. As Brooks et al. found, a long cemented tibial stem has been shown to carry 23–38 % of the axial load and thus reduce the stresses about the periarticular bone or augments [4]. Similarly, extra-articular nonunions and malunion corrections can also be bypassed with stemmed components (see Fig. 4.4). In unique cases, standard revision implants may not provide appropriate reconstruction. Distal femoral replacement often offers the best alternative for severe distal

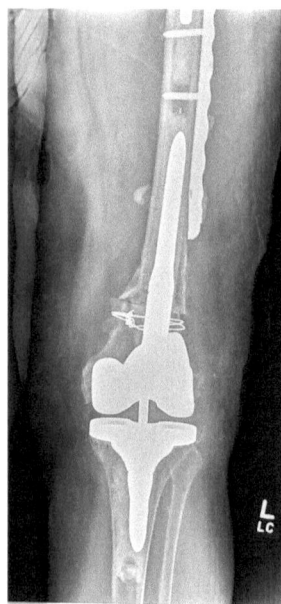

FIG. 4.4. AP radiograph showing a long cemented stem bypassing a distal malunion correction.

femur bone deficiency and allows for immediate weight bearing (see Fig. 4.5).

The posttraumatic knee often presents with ligamentous laxity, rigid deformities, and arthrofibrosis that may often require significant releases for ligament balancing and deformity correction. One must be prepared to address instability with constrained varus-valgus implants as we have found that, in this setting, predictable soft tissue balancing is often unachievable. It is important to remember to use the lowest level of constraint that still provides a stable, balanced knee.

4.4   Intraoperative Considerations

In patients with retained hardware that must be partially or completely removed, incision design and soft tissue handling becomes critically important. Surgical principles must be

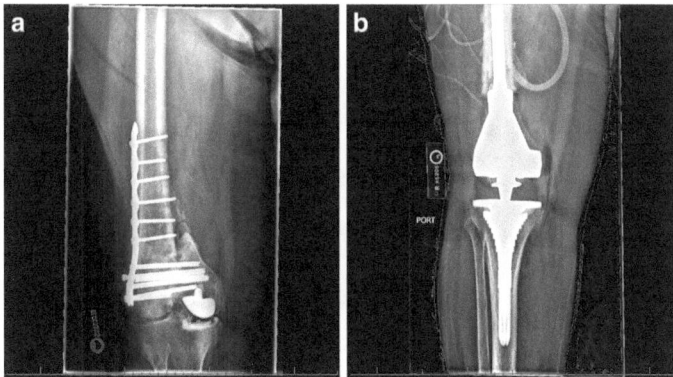

FIG. 4.5. (**a**) AP radiograph showing periprosthetic distal femur fracture with intra-articular extension and compromised bone stock. (**b**) AP radiograph after reconstruction with distal femoral replacement.

respected in order to avoid wound-healing complications. Sharp dissection, full thickness flaps, adequate skin bridges between incisions, avoidance of extensive undermining, and aggressive skin retraction are all part of proper soft tissue handling. In patients with multiple incisions, we recommend use of the most lateral incision to help preserve the dominant, medial, supply to the area [5].

If any doubt arises intraoperatively with regard to the viability of the skin flaps, the operation should end upon hardware removal and the arthroplasty completed in a staged fashion once the soft tissue has healed. Consultation with a plastic surgeon preoperatively may be warranted for certain cases with questionable wound-healing potential, so that adequate coverage can be planned and discussed with the patient.

Posttraumatic knees are often very stiff which makes the surgical exposure difficult. The incidence of intraoperative extensor mechanism disruption has been reported to be as high as 8 % [6]. Therefore, the liberal use of an extensile approach is warranted. Massin et al. reported a need for

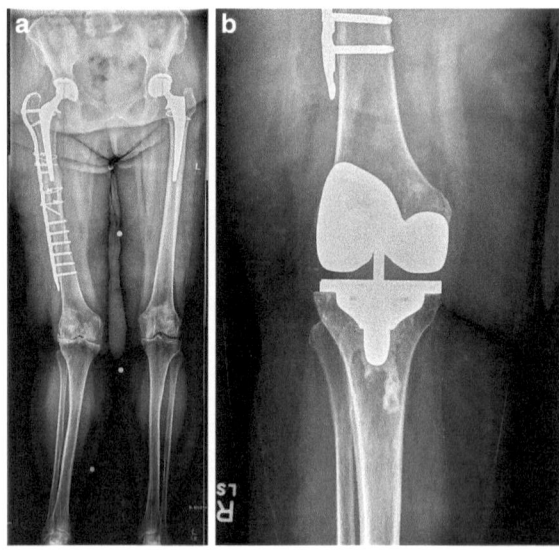

FIG. 4.6. (**a**) Full-length radiograph showing intramedullary hardware preventing use of traditional intramedullary instrumentation requiring use of computer-assisted navigation. (**b**) AP radiograph following CAS total knee arthroplasty.

a tibial tubercle osteotomy in 35 % of patients with posttraumatic arthritis with significant flexion limitations [7]. The authors' preferred extensile approach, when appropriate, is the quadriceps snip.

Another important intraoperative consideration is whether conventional instrumentation can be used effectively in the presence of hardware that violates the intramedullary canal (see Fig. 4.6). Previous reports have shown high midterm aseptic failure rates (26 %) in total knees performed for posttraumatic arthritis knees due to malalignment [8]. Computer navigation is an attractive alternative in order to improve component alignment and avoid significant and unnecessary hardware removal. Not only can computer-assisted surgery (CAS) help navigate intramedullary hardware, but it can also help with extra-articular deformities that make intramedullary guides unreliable. Fehring et al. found that the use of

CAS reliably resulted in proper alignment of the femoral component to within 3° of the mechanical axis in 16 of 17 patients they studied for whom traditional intramedullary guides could not be used [9].

4.5   Results

The goals of arthroplasty in the setting of posttraumatic arthritis with retained hardware are identical to those in an injury-naïve knee, namely restoration of the mechanical axis and creation of a stable joint with appropriately positioned implants. While it is possible to achieve these goals, it is well established such patients are at increased risk of intraoperative and postoperative complications and an inferior clinical outcomes. Weiss et al. reported a 26 % complication rate following total knee arthroplasty after prior tibial plateau fracture including stiffness, wound dehiscence, deep infection, and patellar tendon rupture [6]. Lonner et al. reported a 57 % complication rate following total knee arthroplasty for posttraumatic knees, including aseptic failure, septic failure, patellar tendon rupture, and patellar maltracking [8]. Furthermore, Weiss et al. reported that in patients with a history of femur fracture, only 52 % of their cohort had restoration of limb alignment, correction of the deformity, and ideal component positioning. In their patients with previous tibial plateau fractures, that percentage increased to 77 % [6, 10].

Despite predictable improvements, the functional outcomes of total knee arthroplasty for posttraumatic knees are modest compared to expected improvements after a primary total knee arthroplasty for the typical osteoarthritic patient. Lonner et al. reported only 58 % good to excellent functional scores [8] while Weiss et al. reported good to excellent results in 77 %, fair in 11 %, and poor in 11 % in their series [10]. The biggest gains in the clinical scores appear to be in pain relief.

Though TKAs in the posttraumatic knee with retained hardware are a suitable option to improve function and pain, they require a thorough understanding of the surgical pitfalls.

The reconstruction is technically demanding and associated with a higher complication and reoperation rate. Proper surgical planning and execution must be paired with a preoperative discussion about realistic postoperative outcomes with the patient.

References

1. Honkonen SE. Degenerative arthritis after tibial plateau fractures. J Orthop Trauma. 1995;9:273–7.
2. Suzuki G, et al. Previous fracture surgery is a major risk factor of infection after total knee arthroplasty. Knee Surg Sports Traumatol Arthrosc. 2011;19(12):2040–4.
3. Klatte TO, Schneider MM, Citak M. Infection rates in patients undergoing primary knee arthroplasty with pre-existing proposed if fixation-devices. Knee. 2013;20(3):177–80.
4. Brooks PJ, Walker PS, Scott RD. Tibial component fixation in deficient tibial bone stock. Clin Orthop Relat Res. 1984;184:302–8.
5. Colombel M, Mariz Y, et al. Arterial and lymphatic supply of the knee integuments. Surg Radiol Anat. 1998;20(1):35–40.
6. Weiss NG, Parvizi J, Trousdale RT, et al. Total knee arthroplasty in patients with a prior fracture of the tibial plateau. J Bone Joint Surg. 2003;85-A(2):218–21.
7. Massin P. Total knee replacement in post-traumatic arthritic knees with limitation of flexion. Orthop Traumatol Surg Res. 2011;97(1):28–33.
8. Lonner JH, Pedlow FX, Siliski JM. Total knee arthroplasty for post-traumatic arthrosis. J Arthroplasty. 1999;14(8):969–75.
9. Fehring Thomas K, et al. When computer-assisted knee replacement is the best alternative. Clin Orthop Relat Res. 2006;452:132–6.
10. Weiss NG, Parvizi J, et al. Total knee arthroplasty in post-traumatic arthrosis. J Arthroplast. 2003;18(3):23–6.

Chapter 5
Complex Primary Total Knee Arthroplasty: Management of Extra-articular Deformity

Lucas Armstrong and William A. Jiranek

5.1 Case Presentation

A 70-year-old female who sustained an osteoporotic proximal tibia fracture approximately 5 years prior to presentation. This was treated with an ORIF that failed and fixation was revised with an intramedullary nail. The fracture healed with a varus malunion. She subsequently developed posttraumatic arthritis of her left knee. She has failed comprehensive conservative management of her knee arthritis.

5.1.1 Diagnosis/Assessment

Physical exam revealed an antalgic gait favoring the left side, with a mild varus thrust. There was minimal visible varus deformity of the tibia but the patient had an overall varus alignment of bilateral lower extremities, left much greater than the right. She had a well-healed midline incision over

L. Armstrong, MD (✉)
McLean County Orthopedics, Ltd., Bloomington, IL, USA
e-mail: armstrong.luke77@gmail.com

W.A. Jiranek, MD
Department of Orthopedic Surgery, VCU Health System, Richmond, VA, USA

© Springer International Publishing Switzerland 2015   55
B.D. Springer and B.M. Curtin (eds.), *Complex Primary and Revision Total Knee Arthroplasty: A Clinical Casebook*, DOI 10.1007/978-3-319-18350-3_5

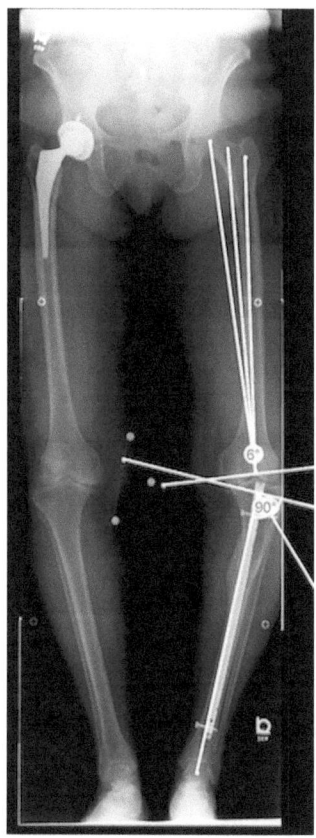

Fɪɢ. 5.1. Preoperative long-standing film showing preoperative plan.

her left knee, no erythema or drainage, and no knee effusion. Her left knee range of motion was 0–110° with no extensor lag. The left knee deformity is correctable and her knee is ligamentously stable. Radiographs reveal an IM nail in her left tibia, with a broken proximal locking screw, varus malunion of the proximal tibia, Kellgren-Lawrence stage 4 medial compartment osteoarthritis, patellofemoral arthritis, and patella baja (Figs. 5.1 and 5.2). Due to previous surgery

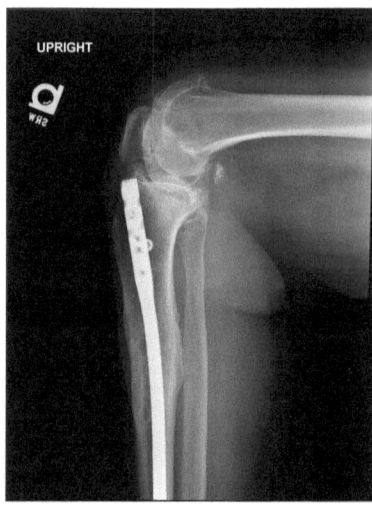

FIG. 5.2. Preoperative lateral film.

and the patient report of a nonunion, she was screened for infection with an ESR and CRP and scheduled for left total knee arthroplasty.

5.1.2 Management

Patient underwent left lower extremity hardware removal and total knee arthroplasty in a single surgery. The varus deformity was significant and the superficial MCL was released in order to balance the knee. A larger than normal polyethylene insert was needed to fill the flexion and extension gaps after the aggressive medial release. We were prepared to increase the constraint, but this was not necessary. The deformity was corrected intra-articularly without the use of computer navigation or the requirement for extra-articular correction.

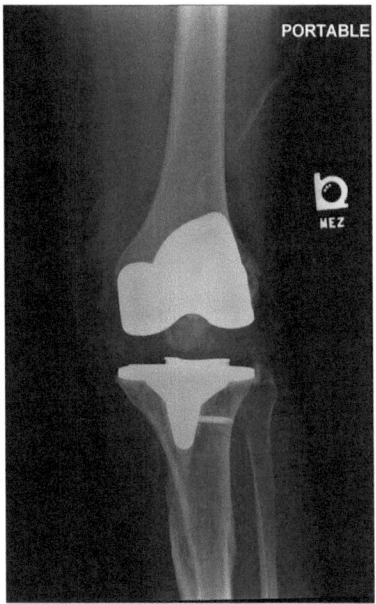

Fig. 5.3. Postoperative AP film showing intra-articular correction.

5.1.3   Outcome

The patient recovered uneventfully following our standard TKA postoperative protocol. She is doing well with a ligamentously stable knee and a postoperative range of motion of 0–105° (Figs. 5.3 and 5.4).

5.2   Literature Review

Lower extremity extra-articular deformity can occur due to prior trauma, surgery, metabolic bone disease, or congenital malformations. It can be complicated by many things, such as previously placed hardware and prior incisions. These interfere with instrumentation and alter landmarks. Long-standing deformity leads to soft tissue contractures requiring releases.

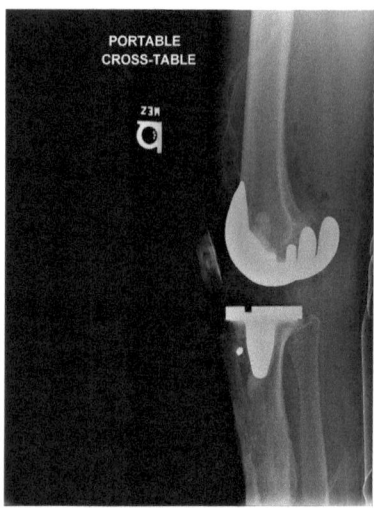

F<small>IG</small>. 5.4. Postoperative lateral film.

The goals of performing a TKA in a person with extra-articular deformity are the same as those for a TKA with the diagnosis of idiopathic osteoarthritis. One needs to establish a neutral mechanical axis and a ligamentously balanced and stable knee throughout a functional arc of motion. In general, deformities of the femur are more difficult to deal with than deformities of the tibia due to the intramedullary instrumentation of the femur used with conventional instrumentation.

When faced with these challenging cases, there are a few basic principles that need to be addressed. Most importantly the patient needs to be counseled on the increased risk of complications and decreased functional outcomes of these surgeries compared to primary cases. Full-length extremity films need to be obtained to preoperatively plan for deformity correction and a CT may be considered to evaluate rotational deformity. Indolent infection should be ruled out with screening labs (ESR and C-reactive protein) and possible joint aspiration if serologies are elevated or there is a high clinical suspicion for infection. Hardware removal does not need to be staged with the exception of a diagnosed infection and only the hardware that interferes with surgery should be removed. If possible, previous incisions should be used and old incisions should be crossed at right angles.

The first decision that needs to be made is if the deformity is correctable with intra-articular bony cuts and ligamentous releases or is an extra-articular correction required. The amount of correction needed is positively correlated to the severity of the deformity and inversely correlated to the distance of the deformity from the joint line [1]. A small deformity of the proximal femur is more easily corrected than a large deformity of the distal femur. Intra-articular correction is the most desirable scenario because it is more familiar to the surgeon and more efficient. A previous study has determined that intra-articular correction is possible if the bony resection is <20° in the femoral coronal plane, <25° in the femoral sagittal plane, and <30° in the tibial coronal plane [2]. Most importantly however, these resections should not compromise the insertions of the collateral ligaments. Intra-articular correction also eliminates problems associated with an osteotomy, which are discussed later. The decision of intra vs. extra-articular correction is based on the amount of correction desired and determined on the full-length standing hip-knee-ankle film. If the amount of bony resection will compromise the insertions of the collateral ligaments, then an extra-articular osteotomy is necessary.

Extra-articular osteotomies allow a larger correction but bring about the possibilities of osteotomy nonunion and decreased weight-bearing status that may interfere with rehabilitation after TKA. Osteotomies may also require additional incisions in an already poor soft tissue envelope. The traditional operative procedure is a two-stage approach of osteotomy and fixation followed by TKA after the osteotomy has healed (Figs. 5.5, 5.6, 5.7, 5.8, 5.9, and 5.10). Some surgeons have attempted a one-stage surgery with intraoperative computer navigation with mixed results [3–5]. Older studies warn that simultaneous surgery produces inferior outcomes [6, 7]. Most of these surgeries were performed

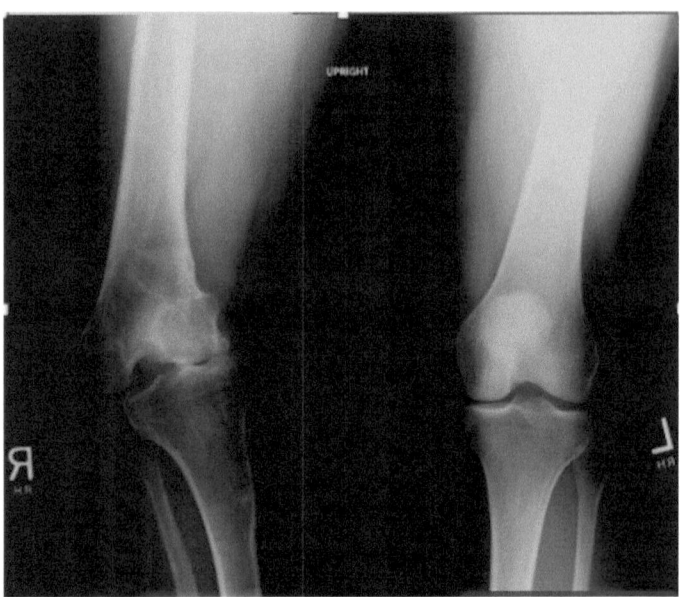

FIG. 5.5. Preoperative AP film showing significant coronal plane deformity of both femur and tibia.

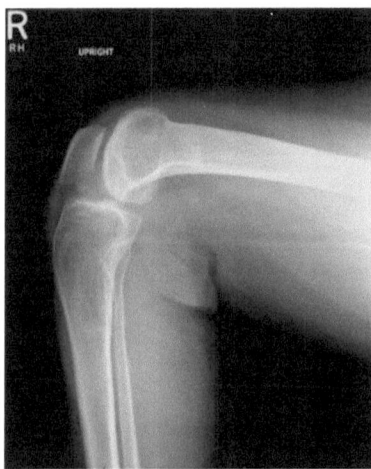

FIG. 5.6. Preoperative lateral film showing minimal sagittal plane deformity.

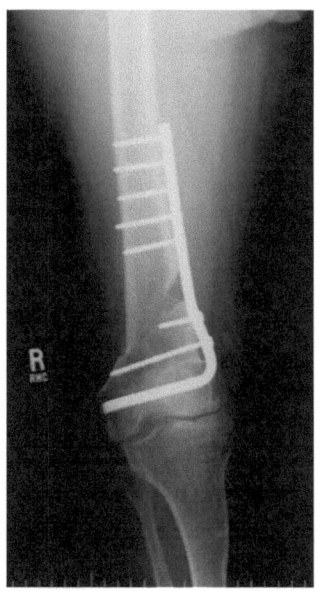

FIG. 5.7. Postoperative AP film showing medial opening wedge osteotomy.

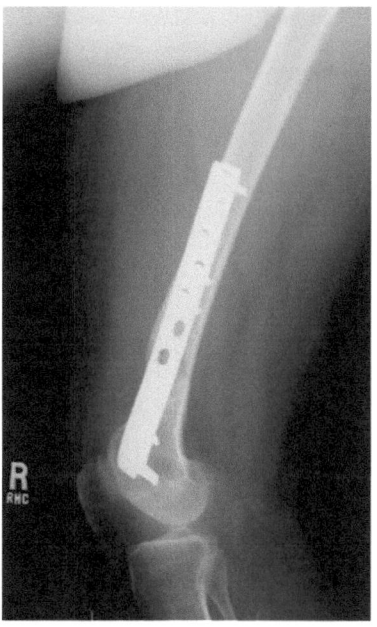

FIG. 5.8. Postoperative lateral film of osteotomy.

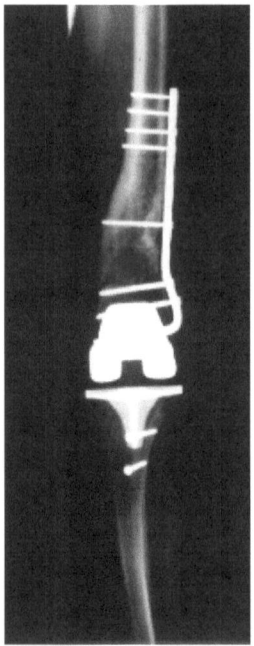

FIG. 5.9. Postoperative AP film showing TKA approximately 5 years after osteotomy.

without computer navigation assistance or stemmed implants. One computer-assisted study evaluating a subset of procedures that required a simultaneous osteotomy (3/40 TKAs) showed no outcome differences or increase in complications [3]. Worse outcomes and increased complications have been shown when simultaneous surgery is performed without navigation [4].

At times hardware is already placed due to previous fracture fixation. Removing the hardware from a united distal femur or proximal tibia fracture would create stress risers from screw tracts and may necessitate additional incisions for hardware removal. The femoral canal may be ablated due to fracture healing making the placement of intramedullary instrumentation difficult. Only the hardware that interferes

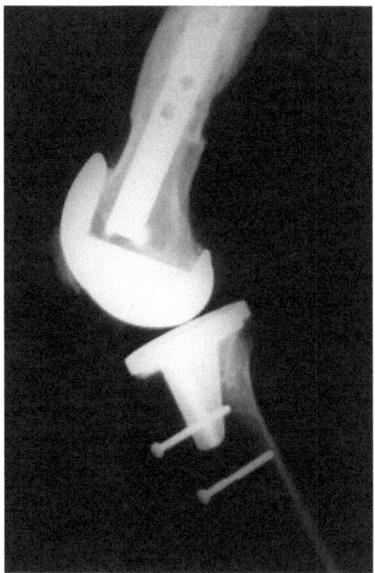

Fɪɢ. 5.10. Postoperative lateral film showing TKA.

with component placement should be removed. For instance, the distal screws in a proximal tibial plate and the plate itself may be left in place to avoid creating a stress riser.

In the setting of previous hardware placement (especially in the femur) or a circuitous femoral canal, computer-assisted navigation can be utilized. Multiple studies and meta-analyses show that navigation improves mechanical alignment in routine TKA vs. conventional instrumentation [8–10]. This technology negates the need for hardware removal or intra-medullary femoral instrumentation and as a result is extremely advantageous in the setting of extra-articular deformity. When no osteotomy is required, the surgical technique is very similar for computer-assisted primary TKA. If an osteotomy is performed, the femoral array should be placed proximal to the osteotomy and be unicortical to avoid hardware or stemmed components [11]. There have been no direct outcome studies comparing computer-navigated TKA with conventional instrumentation in the setting of extra-articular deformity, with or without osteotomy. Most case series utilizing computer-assisted navigation have reported very favorable radiographic outcomes with and without osteotomy [3, 12–14]. A few studies also reported improvement in function and pain scores postoperatively [14, 15]. Similarly, one of the most recent studies shows increase in knee range of motion and Knee Society Scores after TKA utilizing intra-articular correction only, without using computer navigation [16].

Similar to computer-assisted navigation, custom-made cutting guides have the advantage of avoiding instrumentation in the femoral canal and the corresponding benefits listed previously. One of the pioneers of this technique states that absolute indications for custom-made cutting guides include extra-articular deformities, retained hardware, and difficulties with intramedullary instrumentation [17]. It is also possible to produce a computer model of the limb post-osteotomy and use this technology in a one-stage surgery. The inherent problem is the actual surgical osteotomy would have to very closely approximate the preoperative model to avoid errors in mechanical alignment and rotation. Another possible limitation is previously placed surgical hardware interfering with the preoperative scan used to produce the computer model. To date there have been no outcome studies using these guides in the setting of extra-articular deformity.

No matter what technology is used to perform the TKA, if the patient had a previous open surgery on the same extremity, it is pertinent to consider the use of antibiotic impregnated bone cement. Hybrid cement fixation of stemmed components has also shown improved survivorship [18]. Extensive preoperative planning cannot be stressed enough.

5.3 Conclusion

TKA in the setting of extra-articular deformity is a challenging problem. The surgical difficulty is much greater than a primary TKA. Exhaustive preoperative planning is imperative for a successful outcome. A critical decision involves whether the deformity can be corrected intra-articularly with the bone cuts and ligamentous releases or require extra-articular correction with an osteotomy. The patient should be warned of increased risks and decreased outcomes as well as screened for indolent infection. The use of computer assistance, especially in the setting of femoral deformity, is extremely valuable.

5.4   Clinical Pearls/Pitfalls

- Patients must be appropriately counseled and screened for infection.
- Intra-articular correction is more familiar to surgeons and eliminates possible complications from osteotomies.
- The closer the deformity is to the involved joint, the more difficult intra-articular correction becomes and often requires extra-articular correction.
- Preoperative planning (obtaining previous operative reports and implant records) is imperative for a successful outcome.
- Hardware removal can be done in the same surgery, with the exception of diagnosed infection.
- Computer-assisted navigation is a valuable tool in the setting of TKA with extra-articular deformity.

References

1. Wolff AM, Hungerford DS, Pepe CL. The effect of extraarticular varus and valgus deformity on total knee arthroplasty. Clin Orthop Relat Res. 1991;271(Oct):35–51.
2. Wang JW, Wang CJ. Total knee arthroplasty for arthritis of the knee with extra-articular deformity. J Bone Joint Surg Am. 2002;84-A(10):1769–74.
3. Mullaji A, Shetty GM. Computer-assisted total knee arthroplasty for arthritis with extra-articular deformity. J Arthroplasty. 2009;24(8):1164–9.

4. Papadopoulos EC, Parvizi J, Lai CH, Lewallen DG. Total knee arthroplasty following prior distal femoral fracture. Knee. 2002;9(4):267–74.
5. Lonner JH, Siliski JM, Lotke PA. Simultaneous femoral osteotomy and total knee arthroplasty for treatment of osteoarthritis associated with severe extra-articular deformity. J Bone Joint Surg Am. 2000;82(3):342–8.
6. Cameron HU, Welsh RP. Potential complications of total knee replacement following tibial osteotomy. Orthop Rev. 2004; 17(1):39–43.
7. Roffi RP, Merritt PO. Total knee replacement after fractures about the knee. Orthop Rev. 1989;19(7):614–20.
8. Chauhan SK, Scott RG, Breidal W, et al. Computer-assisted knee arthroplasty versus a conventional jig-based technique: a randomized, prospective trial. J Bone Joint Surg (Br). 2004; 86-B(3):372–7.
9. Chin PL, Yang KY, Yeo SF, Lo NN. Randomized control trial comparing radiographic total knee arthroplasty implant placement using computer navigation versus conventional technique. J Arthroplasty. 2005;20(5):618–26.
10. Mason JB, Fehring TK, Estok R, Banal D, Fahrbach K. Meta-analysis of alignment outcomes in computer-assisted total knee arthroplasty surgery. J Arthroplasty. 2007;22(8):1097–106.
11. Mason JB, Fehring TK. Management of extra-articular deformity in total knee arthroplasty with navigation. In: Norman Scott W, editor. Insall& Scott surgery of the knee. 5th ed. Philadelphia: Elsevier; 2012. p. p1232–9.
12. Klein GR, Austin MS, SMith EB, Hozack WJ. Total knee arthroplasty using computer-assisted navigation in patients with deformities of the femur and tibia. J Arthroplasty. 2006;21(2):284–8.
13. Fehring TK, Mason JB, Moskal J, Pollack DC, Mann J, Williams VJ. When computer-assisted knee replacement is the best alternative. Clin Orthop Relat Res. 2006;452(Nov):132–6.
14. Bottros J, Klika AK, Lee HH, Polousky J, Barsoum WK. The use of navigation in total knee arthroplasty for patients with extra-articular deformity. J Arthroplasty. 2008;23(1):74–8.
15. Kim K, Ramteke AA, Bae DK. Navigation-assisted minimal invasive total knee arthroplasty in patients with extra-articular femoral deformity. J Arthroplasty. 2010;25(4):658.e17–22.
16. Marczk D, Snyder M, Sibiński M, et al. One-stage total knee arthroplasty with pre-existing fracture deformity: post fracture total knee arthroplasty. J Arthroplasty. 2014;29(11):2104–8.

17. Hafez M. Custom-made cutting guides for total knee arthroplasty. In: Norman Scott W, editor. Insall& Scott surgery of the knee. 5th ed. Philadelphia: Elsevier; 2012. p. 1240–54.
18. Gofton WT, Tsigara H, Butler RA, Patterson JJ, Barrack RL, Rorabeck CH. Revision total knee arthroplasty: fixation with modular stems. Clin Orthop Relat Res. 2002;404:158–68.

Chapter 6
Complex Primary Total Knee Arthroplasty: Management of Complex Skin Incisions

Jeremy M. Gililland and Lucas A. Anderson

6.1 Case Presentation

A 48-year-old Caucasian female presented with a lifelong history of right lower extremity deformity related to extensive hemangiomas and right knee pain. She had developed several years of progressive varus deformity and pain related to degenerative arthritis of the left knee (Fig. 6.1). She had failed conservative interventions and was referred for discussion of total knee arthroplasty.

The patient was born with a large cavernous hemangioma of the right lower extremity involving the entirety of the thigh, lateral and anterior aspect of the knee and extending to the proximal tibia. She had previous treatment with radiation therapy and seven surgical procedures including a cross-leg flap from the posterior calf of the left leg to provide skin coverage over the anterior right knee. This resulted in a large, bulbous flap approximately 15 cm in diameter (Fig. 6.2). As a result of her radiation therapy, extensive dense scar extended from the lateral hip down to the lateral calf. At the level of the knee, this scar tissue was primarily posterolaterally located and was associated with a 20° hard flexion contracture of the

J.M. Gililland, MD (✉) • L.A. Anderson, MD
University of Utah, Salt Lake City, UT, USA
e-mail: jeremy.gililland@hsc.utah.edu

© Springer International Publishing Switzerland 2015   69
B.D. Springer and B.M. Curtin (eds.), *Complex Primary and Revision Total Knee Arthroplasty: A Clinical Casebook*,
DOI 10.1007/978-3-319-18350-3_6

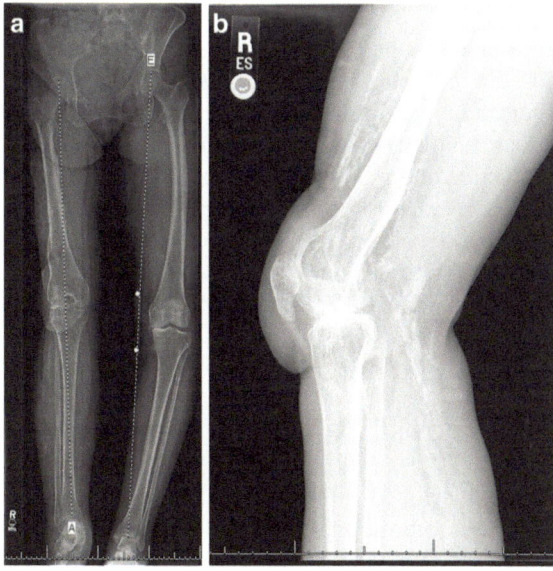

FIG. 6.1. (**a**) Long-standing radiograph of bilateral knee osteoarthritis. (**b**) Preoperative lateral radiograph of right knee with distal femoral malunion.

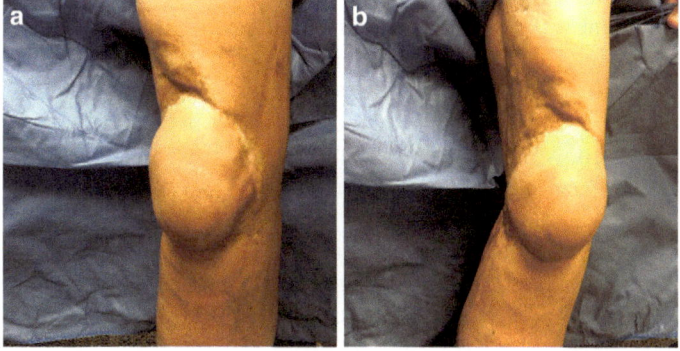

FIG. 6.2. (**a, b**) Photographs of lateral and posterolateral external scarring and prior cross-leg flap to anterior right knee.

knee (Fig. 6.2b). In the distribution of this scar tissue, the patient had developed severe hypersensitivity that had been diagnosed as complex regional pain syndrome (CRPS).

Other than her musculoskeletal issues, the patient was healthy and had a BMI of 28. She had neutral alignment of the right knee and a 20° flexion contracture (ROM from 20 to 50°). There was no opening laterally with varus stress as the knee had developed a severe posterolateral based external scar contracture. There was an intact extensor mechanism and she had intact sensation and palpable pulses in the right foot.

6.2   Diagnosis/Evaluation

Initially, we discussed with this patient the surgical options of above knee amputation, fusion, and arthroplasty. We had the patient meet with several local amputation patients, with prosthetists, and with our orthopedic oncology partners for a second opinion. We met with the patient several times over a 7-month period while she was investigating her surgical options. We counseled her that there was considerable risk of worsening her pre-existing complex regional pain syndrome and that flap and skin necrosis may occur. We discussed with her that if her soft tissue necrosis did occur, this may lead to the need for free flap coverage or even above knee amputation if she were to develop periprosthetic joint infection. After extensive informed consent, the patient elected to proceed with total knee arthroplasty with the soft tissue management plan of a midline incision through her existing cross-leg flap.

A preoperative consultation with a plastic surgeon was obtained to evaluate the tissues about the knee and vascular surgeons to evaluate the status of the large hemangiomas in the right lower extremity. An MRI was performed showing diffuse venous vascular malformation extending from the right hemipelvis to below the knee. There were extensive hemangiomas in the anterior and posterior right thigh compartments and very mild osseous involvement in the mid

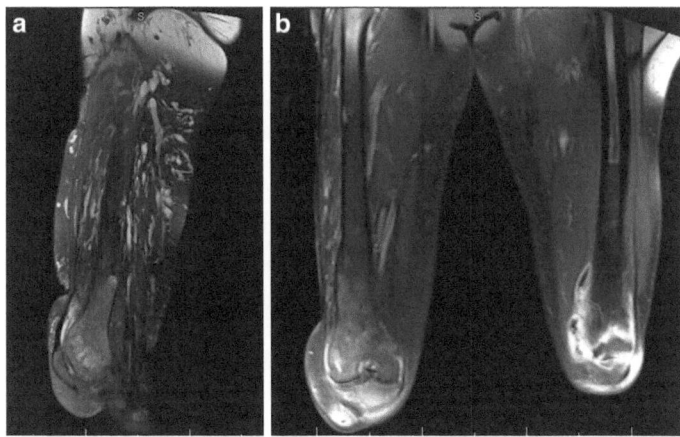

Fɪɢ. 6.3. Sagittal (**a**) and coronal (**b**) MRI imaging of vascular malformations of right thigh and periarticular region.

femoral shaft (Fig. 6.3). Intra-articularly, there was only suprapatellar pouch involvement with minimal involvement of the lateral knee or articular surfaces.

The preoperative evaluation with the vascular surgeons revealed that since the majority of the vascular malformations were in the posterior thigh and did not involve the articular surfaces of the knee, that total knee arthroplasty would be reasonable. The plastic surgeons advised that with a cross-leg flap there was no specific pedicle to preserve and thus recommended a longitudinal full thickness incision through the midline of this flap with elevation of full thickness subfascial flaps medial and lateral. We discussed lifting the flap from the lateral most aspect to follow the general principle of using prior lateral based incisions. However, as this knee had undergone prior skin grafting and irradiation, there was abundant scar along the interface between the flap and lateral skin. Additionally we were concerned that if we had to elevate the entire flap from the lateral side that we may disturb the blood supply to the majority of the flap and lose our coverage over the entire anterior knee.

6.3   Management and Treatment Options of Complex Skin Issues

Preoperative evaluation of the TKA patient should always involve a close examination of the soft tissues. The presence of prior incisions or scarring should prompt a discussion of prior surgical interventions or trauma and when they occurred. It is often felt that old incisions can be ignored in the setting of TKA; however, if any prior longitudinal incision is ignored, the consequences can be devastating as seen in the clinical photos in Fig. 6.4 of a patient 6 weeks after a new medial incision was made in the setting of an ignored 20 years old lateral based incision. The majority of blood supply to the anterior skin around the knee comes from terminal branches of a peripatellar anastomotic ring of arteries in the subcutaneous fascia, most of which enters from the medial side. Therefore, flap formation over the anterior knee should be performed deep to the subcutaneous fascia to avoid disrupting this blood supply. If multiple prior longitudinal incisions exist, the lateral most incision should be utilized whenever possible so as to minimize the size of vulnerable lateral flap. If prior oblique, or transverse incisions exist, these can most safely be approached at 90° angles to limit the risk of necrosis in the corners where these incisions meet. In general, angles of less than 60° between a prior oblique incision and the new proposed incision should be avoided.

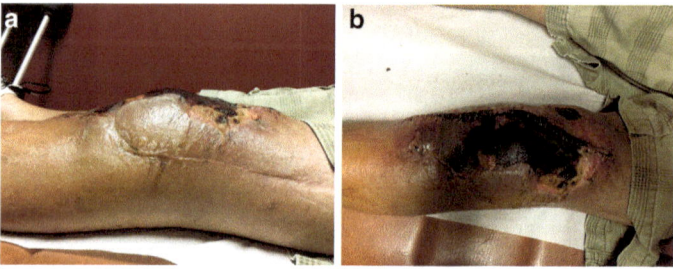

Fig. 6.4. (**a, b**) Photographs of knee with skin necrosis after midline incision made adjacent to prior lateral incision.

When performing incisions on knees with prior flaps, the source of blood supply needs to be considered. Preoperatively, the type of prior flaps and their potential pedicles should be investigated through discussion with plastic surgeons, reading prior operative reports, and possible advanced imaging to assess blood supply to the flap.

Soft tissue expanders may be indicated if periarticular skin is compromised by multiple prior crossing incisions, flaps, or severe deformity preventing skin mobilization and coverage after the reconstruction is performed. Expanders are generally utilized for a period of 8–10 weeks with injection of saline into a subdermal port and have yielded favorable long-term results [1]. Typically, patients with prior skin graft, irradiated tissue, or densely adherent scar tissue are contraindicated for soft tissue expansion and may require flap coverage prior to their arthroplasty procedure. In our case, our patient did have a prior flap and we considered using a soft tissue expander preoperatively, but due to the fact that she also had some areas of skin grafting, irradiated tissues, and adherent scar tissue, we elected to avoid expansion.

Historically, sham incisions were utilized to determine viability of soft tissues to heal prior to implantation of components. Planned incisions were performed down to the retinaculum and then closed and allowed to heal for several weeks to evaluate the healing potential of the tissue. Unfortunately, if the sham incision fails to heal, then flap coverage may be necessary and this technique has thus fallen out of favor.

6.4   Surgical Technique

We started this case without inflation of the tourniquet so that we could better visualize any superficial hemangiomas and to better assess the bleeding in our cross-leg flap as we performed the superficial dissection. Our plastic surgery team assisted intraoperatively with exposure in this case; the skin incision was an anterior midline incision directly through the cross-leg flap and there was good bleeding from both the medial and lateral flap edges. Full thickness flaps were developed with attached subcutaneous fascia beneath permitting exposure for a standard medial parapatellar arthrotomy. Nylon suture was used to maintain the dermal, subcutaneous and subcutaneous fascial layers as one flap; these were sutured to wet laps on each side and then sutured back and secured to the skin to permit retraction without trauma from rigid retractors and to prevent drying out of the flaps.

The tourniquet was then inflated and the medial parapatellar arthrotomy was performed. As predicted by the pre-op MRI, we did encounter several small hemangiomas in the region of the suprapatellar pouch and superficial soft tissues proximal to the patella and these were ligated without significant bleeding. The vascular surgery team was available should large cavernous hemangiomas be encountered.

Severely limited flexion necessitated a quadriceps snip in order to adequately flex the knee for exposure. We then performed a gap-balanced total knee arthroplasty starting with a computer-navigated distal femoral cut due to the vascular abnormalities involving the femoral bone and her prior malunited distal femur fracture. Due to severe posterolateral external soft tissue scar contractures the posterolateral corner, IT band, and LCL were released and we still had significant posterolateral tightness in extension necessitating a varus-valgus constrained polyethylene liner (Fig. 6.5). Motion after re-approximation of the quad snip and release of the tourniquet was 10–70°

Our plastic surgery colleagues then assisted with superficial closure in layers after arthrotomy closure. A hemovac drain deep to the arthrotomy closure and a flat JP drain superficial to the arthrotomy layer were placed. Both the medial and lateral aspects of the cross-leg flap were found to have adequate capillary refill and bleeding skin edges at the time of closure. The knee was placed into a bulky dressing and knee immobilizer. The plastic surgeon emphasized maximizing soft tissue perfusion postoperatively by keeping the patient's room warm and avoiding caffeine, cooling blankets, constrictive ace wraps, and TED hose.

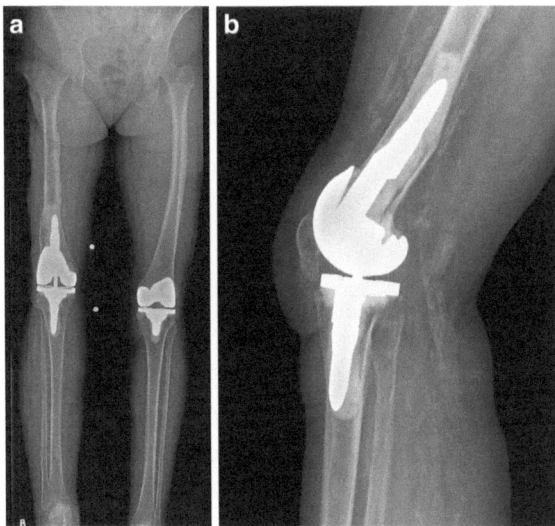

Fig. 6.5. (**a**, **b**) Postoperative radiographs of right TKA showing stemmed constrained components in good alignment.

6.5   Outcome

Postoperatively, the patient had excellent pain relief and noted an improved sense of stability. On post-op day 2, the lateral aspect of the cross-leg flap developed some blistering and epidermolysis while some skin edge necrosis developed along the incision edges at the distal aspect of the cross-leg flap. The plastics team felt that an incisional wound VAC over the skin incision and hyperbaric oxygen therapy would aid in vascularization of these areas. An incisional wound VAC was placed over the distal incision and this was left in place for approximately 10 days. The patient received hyperbaric oxygen treatments over the next 6 weeks. Dry eschars formed in the lateral skin where the epidermolysis had occurred and along the edges of the skin incision without any gross evidence of infection (Fig. 6.6). There was no drainage and the patient did not have any increasing pain.

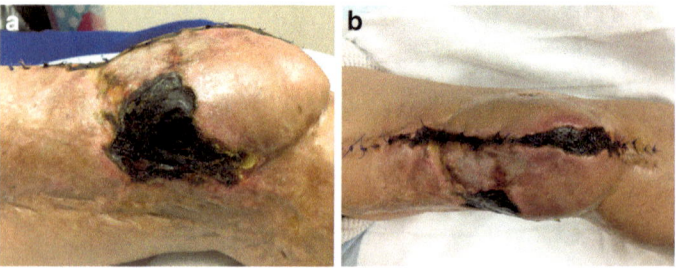

FIG. 6.6. (**a**, **b**) Photographs showing dry eschar formation 1 month after surgery.

We left these dry eschars in place and allowed the patient to begin gentle range of motion limited to about 45° of flexion after 4 weeks post-op. The patient had complete normalization of her inflammatory markers by 4 weeks post-op (ESR 10, CRP 0.2). Healthy granulation tissue developed beneath these eschars and the patient went on to successful wound healing.

6.6 Literature Review

As is highlighted with this complex case, thorough preoperative planning and a multidisciplinary team approach to both the intraoperative and postoperative care are often necessary to successfully perform an arthroplasty in knees with difficult skin or prior incisions. Inadequate preparation can lead to soft tissue necrosis, need for soft tissue coverage procedures, infection, extensor mechanism disruption, and possibly the need for amputation. As already emphasized, in difficult soft tissue cases it is essential to carefully plan out the skin incision to be used and to understand when soft tissue expansion may be necessary.

The use of soft tissue expanders has shown successful long-term results in knees at risk for problematic wound healing. In a series of 28 knee arthroplasties after soft tissue expansion with mean follow-up of almost 3 years, Manifold et al.

found no major wound complications after the total knee arthroplasties and average Knee Society Score of 83.7 [1]. They did find 21 % minor wound complications during the expansions and 18 % after the arthroplasties. One major wound complication of skin necrosis did occur during expansion in a patient with history of prior radiation to the skin. This patient required skin grafting and did not go on to subsequent arthroplasty.

If skin necrosis does occur postoperatively, a variety of techniques exist to aid in coverage; however avoiding soft tissue complications in the first place is ideal. Most of the knee can be covered with either a medial or lateral gastrocnemius muscle rotation flap. However, free muscle flap coverage may need to be considered if coverage needs to be obtained proximal to the patella. The successful use of medial gastrocnemius rotation flaps and free flaps for prophylactic treatment of adherent skin and scar to the underlying bone prior to performing primary total knee arthroplasty has been described [2]. When skin necrosis does occur after total knee arthroplasty, prompt soft tissue coverage to prevent development of deep infection is often necessary. Medial gastrocnemius flaps are often the workhorse in providing coverage for skin necrosis over the patella and patellar tendon and these have shown good clinical success [3]. Necrosis overlying the patellar tendon usually necessitates flap coverage to avoid infection to the underlying patellar tendon, whereas necrosis over the patella itself can occasionally be successfully treated with local wound care and skin grafting [4]. Skin necrosis that develops proximal to the patella may necessitate free flap or fasciocutaneous flap coverage. More recently, the distally based pedicled gracilis flap has been described to successfully treat superolateral skin defects after TKA where free flap coverage would have traditionally been recommended [5].

As discussed in this case, hyperbaric oxygen therapy has been successfully utilized for the salvage of necrotic skin or flaps and prevention of deep infection in the plastic surgery literature [6]. In a swine model, hyperbaric oxygen therapy led to significant enhancement of skin flap survival [7]. While not described in the arthroplasty setting, this has been successfully utilized to salvage a necrotic flap in breast reconstruction procedures with underlying silicon implants [8].

6.7 Clinical Pearls/Pitfalls

- Carefully consider all skin and soft tissue vulnerabilities in TKA preoperative planning.
- Understanding unique and typical vascular anatomy is key to preserving blood supply to native skin and any prior flap coverage.
- Skin flap formation over the anterior knee should be performed deep to the subcutaneous fascia to avoid disrupting the blood supply.
- If multiple prior longitudinal incisions exist, the lateral most incision should be utilized whenever possible.
- In general, angles of less than 60° between a prior oblique incision and the new proposed incision should be avoided.
- Soft tissue expanders may be indicated if periarticular skin is compromised by multiple prior crossing incisions, flaps, or severe deformity preventing skin mobilization.
- There should be a low threshold to utilize a multidisciplinary team to help co-manage difficult soft tissues, including plastic surgery and vascular surgery.

References

1. Manifold SG, Cushner FD, Craig-Scott S, Scott WN. Long-term results of total knee arthroplasty after the use of soft tissue expanders. Clin Orthop Relat Res. 2000;380:133–9. PubMed English.
2. Markovich GD, Dorr LD, Klein NE, McPherson EJ, Vince KG. Muscle flaps in total knee arthroplasty. Clin Orthop Relat Res. 1995;321:122–30. PubMed English.
3. Ries MD, Bozic KJ. Medial gastrocnemius flap coverage for treatment of skin necrosis after total knee arthroplasty. Clin Orthop Relat Res. 2006;446:186–92. PubMed English.

4. Ries MD. Skin necrosis after total knee arthroplasty. J Arthroplasty. 2002;17(4 Suppl 1):74–7. PubMed English.
5. Mitsala G, Varey AHR, O'Neill JK, Chapman TW, Khan U. The distally pedicled gracilis flap for salvage of complex knee wounds. Injury. 2014;45(11):1776–81. PubMed English.
6. Roje Z, Roje Z, Eterović D, Druzijanić N, Petrićević A, Roje T, et al. Influence of adjuvant hyperbaric oxygen therapy on short-term complications during surgical reconstruction of upper and lower extremity war injuries: retrospective cohort study. Croat Med J. 2008;49(2):224–32. PubMed Pubmed Central PMCID: PMC2359875. English.
7. Pellitteri PK, Kennedy TL, Youn BA. The influence of intensive hyperbaric oxygen therapy on skin flap survival in a swine model. Arch Otolaryngol Head Neck Surg. 1992;118(10):1050–4. PubMed English.
8. Mermans JF, Tuinder S, von Meyenfeldt MF, van der Hulst RRWJ. Hyperbaric oxygen treatment for skin flap necrosis after a mastectomy: a case study. Undersea Hyperb Med. 2012;39(3):719–23. PubMed English.

Chapter 7
Periprosthetic Infection: Management of Early Postoperative Infection

Craig J. Della Valle and Erdan Kayupov

7.1 Case Presentation

A 54-year-old male with a past medical history significant for hepatic failure secondary to alcohol abuse presented with end-stage degenerative joint disease of the knee that had failed nonoperative treatment. His BMI was 32 and other medical comorbidities included hypertension and hypercholesterolemia. As part of his preoperative education, it was explained to him that given his hepatic failure, he was at higher risk for postoperative complications [1]. The patient was seen by his hepatologist in addition to a specialist in internal medicine preoperatively for optimization prior to total knee arthroplasty (TKA).

The patient underwent a cemented, cruciate retaining TKA with antibiotic loaded cement (used by the author selectively in patients felt to be at higher risk for periprosthetic joint infection), and his immediate postoperative course was uncomplicated. He was discharged to home on postoperative day number three. The patient presented on

C.J. Della Valle, MD (✉) • E. Kayupov, MSE
Rush University Medical Center, Chicago, IL, USA
e-mail: craigdv@yahoo.com

© Springer International Publishing Switzerland 2015
B.D. Springer and B.M. Curtin (eds.), *Complex Primary and Revision Total Knee Arthroplasty: A Clinical Casebook*, DOI 10.1007/978-3-319-18350-3_7

81

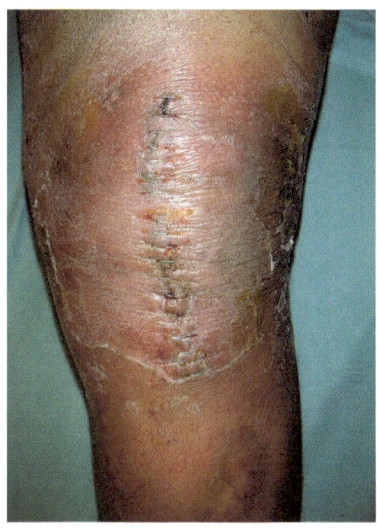

FIG. 7.1. Clinical appearance of the wound on postoperative day 19.

postoperative day 19 with concerns regarding erythema around the incision (Fig. 7.1). He denied any constitutional symptoms or wound drainage.

7.2   Diagnosis

In some cases the diagnosis of a deep periprosthetic joint infection will be straightforward, with purulent drainage from the incision or dehiscence of the wound making the diagnosis clear. In many other cases, however, it is less obvious if the patient has a superficial wound cellulitis that can be managed nonoperatively, if deep PJI exists, or if there is no infection present at all. Normal postoperative pain and inflammation around the surgical site make normal cues to diagnosis less helpful.

In these cases, we have found the serum C-reactive protein (CRP) to be an excellent screening test to determine if an aspiration of the knee is warranted [2]. Specifically, in a study of 146 knees that were evaluated at two centers for deep PJI in the first 6 weeks postoperatively, the serum CRP was found to have excellent overall accuracy at an optimal cutoff value of 95 mg/L (normal, <10 mg/L). Hence, if there is any concern regarding infection in the early postoperative period, we always obtain a serum CRP. If the value is above or anywhere near 100 mg/L (100 being easier to remember than 95), an aspiration of the knee is performed. In general, the aspiration should be performed through an area that is clear of erythema, if possible.

Fluid obtained at the time of aspiration should be sent for a synovial fluid white blood cell (WBC) count and differential to determine the percentage of polymorphonuclear cells, as well as for culture. Prior work from our center has shown the utility of these tests for the diagnosis of *CHRONIC* PJI with optimal cutoff values of 3,000 WBC/μ[mu]L and 80 % for the differential [3]. However, in the acute postoperative phase, defined as within the first 6 weeks after surgery, the work referenced above [2] suggests optimal synovial WBC count and differential values of approximately 10,000 WBC/μ[mu]L and 90 %, respectively. More specifically, the data suggested an even higher cutoff value of 27,800 WBC/μ[mu]L to optimize specificity (good rule in test) and 10,700 WBC/μ[mu]L to optimize sensitivity (good rule out test). In practice I prefer to use the lower threshold number of 10,000 WBC/μ[mu]L. Thus, synovial fluid white blood cell counts below 10,000 WBC/μ[mu]L are considered as not infected, while values above are deemed infected, particularly if the differential is greater than 90 % polymorphonuclear cells. Of note, the synovial fluid white blood cell count and differential values actually change over time [4]. However, in my own experience, the majority of patients where there is concern over infection typically present within the first 6 weeks after their surgery. In cases, where the values are equivocal or if the clinician is just not sure, cultures can be observed and a final decision made based upon their result.

To avoid confusion on diagnosis for any infection, it is imperative that antibiotics be withheld until an aspiration of the knee joint is performed [5]. The administration of antibiotics prior to a thorough evaluation for infection, while tempting, can greatly confuse the diagnosis. Not only will the deep culture results potentially be compromised, but also because the effect of antibiotic treatment on the synovial fluid WBC count and differential as well as serum markers of PJI is not well understood. Furthermore, antibiotic administration prior to obtaining synovial fluid for culture is the strongest risk factor for culture negative PJI [6], which typically leads to suboptimal antibiotic treatment as the offending pathogen can no longer be identified or its antibiotic sensitivities determined. This inability to identify the infecting organism or determine antibiotic sensitivities leads to compromises having to be made in order to cover the most likely organism as opposed to directly targeting a known infecting organism. Finally, if wound drainage is present, it should *NOT* be cultured as these culture results can often confuse treatment decisions [7].

7.3   Management

Management of deep periprosthetic joint infections should be operative. The most commonly utilized strategy for acute postoperative treatment in North America is irrigation and debridement with an exchange of the modular polyethylene bearing surface. However, reported results in the literature are quite variable, with many contemporary series suggesting failure rates of more than 50 %. Several series have also suggested that infections with staphylococcus aureus [8], especially if resistant to methicillin, do particularly poorly [9]. Hence, in some situations the surgeon might consider removing the implants if the identity of the infecting organism is known to be methicillin-resistant staphylococcus aureus prior to embarking upon operative intervention.

If an irrigation and debridement is chosen for management, it should not be relegated to a junior member of the team, as surgical technique may be important to optimizing results and good judgment is required to ensure an adequate and thorough debridement. First, the skin should be meticulously mechanically debrided prior to prepping and draping to remove any sutures, staples, skin glue, and scabbing. The skin edges must be carefully handled to optimize the chances of uneventful wound healing, including raising small but full thickness skin flaps prior to the arthrotomy. Next, the debridement should include a stepwise and thorough anterior synovectomy and exchange of the modular polyethylene liner. Liner trials must be available to ensure the correct size is inserted. In many cases the optimal size liner is somewhat thicker than the original, while in some other cases the surgeon may decide a thinner insert is better.

Next, a posterior synovectomy is performed, but this is admittedly challenging in most situations given the limited exposure posteriorly with implants in place. Then the wound is cleansed with pulsatile lavage, and in our center also soaked with a dilute betadine lavage [10] in an attempt to further decrease bacterial counts in the wound. This is followed by an attempt at mechanical debridement of the metallic surfaces. We typically perform the mechanical debridement with a brush used to cleanse the femoral canal in total hip arthroplasty.

The wound is then again soaked with dilute betadine and cleansed with pulsatile lavage. Prior to insertion of the new polyethylene liner and wound closure, some attempt at re-prepping and draping should be made. This can range from the surgical team changing gloves and using new drapes around the immediate surgical field to a temporary closure of the wound followed by completely breaking down the surgical field and using new gowns, drapes, and a completely new set of instruments. It is still unclear if the former is adequate or if the latter approach will lead to improved results. Wound closure is preferably performed with absorbable, nonbraided suture in layers, taking care to carefully reapproximate the tissue layers including the skin. Some recent data suggest a subcuticular suture is associated with the least compromise of the skin's blood supply [11]. The use of a drain is controversial, but preferred at our center.

Postoperative management includes a team approach comprised of the surgeon, an infectious disease specialist to guide antibiotic treatment, and an internist to optimize medical comorbidities including nutrition. A 6-week course of intravenous antibiotics is routine; however, it is unclear what the optimal duration of therapy is and if intravenous delivery is required. Oral antibiotic "suppressive" therapy for somewhere between 3 months in duration postoperatively to lifelong is routine at our center. However, it is unclear what the optimal duration of "suppressive" therapy is, or if such therapy is even necessary. Some of these decisions will depend on the virulence of the organism, if an oral agent is readily available that matches the organism's sensitivities, the status of the host, and if the patient can tolerate extended oral antibiotic therapy.

Given the less than optimal results of irrigation and debridement, several alternatives to the regimen have been described. One option is a planned "second look" debridement with or without the addition of antibiotic loaded, cement beads that are placed at the time of the first debridement and removed at the second. Others have advocated the use of antibiotic loaded, absorbable calcium sulfate beads; hence, a second operative procedure with its cost and morbidity is avoided. Another reasonable option, particularly if the organism is known prior to surgery and is associated with poor results when treated with isolated irrigation and debridement (e.g., methicillin-resistant Staphylococcus aureus), is to remove the implants and place an antibiotic loaded spacer as the first of a planned two-stage procedure. Finally, some European centers advocated for a one-stage exchange; however, experience with this is limited in North America. If cementless knee devices become more commonly used, a one-stage exchange may become more popular given the ease of implant removal in the early postoperative period prior to osseointegration. Arthroscopy for management of an acute postoperative infection is not recommended, as the modular bearing surface cannot be exchanged and the debridement, although technically possible, may not be adequate. Controversy will persist over the best form of management for acute postoperative infections until more studies, including randomized controlled trials, are performed. Admittedly this will be a challenge given the fortunately low prevalence of this complication.

7.4   Outcome

Given the appearance of the wound, and higher suspicion for infection due to the patient's history of liver dysfunction, a serum CRP was obtained and found to be elevated at 158 mg/dL (normal <10 mg/dL). The knee was subsequently aspirated and the synovial fluid WBC count was 37,000 WBC/μ[mu]L and the differential showed 93 % neutrophils. The patient was brought urgently to the operating room where an irrigation and debridement was performed along with exchange of the modular polyethylene liner; the liner was upsized from a 12 mm liner to a 14 mm liner that had more inherent constraint. Operative cultures grew methicillin-sensitive staphylococcus aureus and he was placed on intravenous cefazolin. Twelve days following the irrigation and debridement, the patient presented with drainage from the wound and the decision was made to return to the operating room where the implants were removed, and an antibiotic loaded spacer was placed as the first part of a planned two-stage exchange.

7.5   Clinical Pearls/Pitfalls

- If an acute postoperative infection is suspected, the surgeon should avoid the temptation to administer any type of antibiotics until an investigation for infection has been performed to rule out a deep periprosthetic joint infection (PJI).
- The serum C-reactive protein has been shown to be an excellent screening test for deep PJI, with an optimal

threshold of approximately 100 mg/dL (normal <10 mg/dL). If the serum CRP is near or above this value, the knee should be aspirated.

- The synovial fluid WBC count and differential are excellent tools for diagnosing acute PJI, albeit at optimal cutoff values that are higher than those used for the diagnosis of chronic PJI. A synovial fluid WBC count of approximately 10,000 WBC/μ[mu]L and a differential of approximately 90 % are the optimal cutoff values.
- While the results of an irrigation and debridement are suboptimal, this remains the most common treatment modality employed given the difficulty in removing well-fixed cemented implants.
- The irrigation and debridement should be done meticulously and carefully to optimize results.
- A multidisciplinary team that includes an infectious disease specialist to guide antibiotic treatment and an internist to optimize nutrition and medical comorbidities is recommended.

References

1. Tiberi 3rd JV, Hansen V, El-Abbadi N, Bedair H. Increased complication rates after hip and knee arthroplasty in patients with cirrhosis of the liver. Clin Orthop Relat Res. 2014;472(9): 2774–8.
2. Bedair H, Ting N, Moric M, Saxena A, Jacovides C, Parvizi J, Della Valle CJ. Mark Coventry Award: diagnosis of infection in the early post-operative period following primary total knee arthroplasty: the utility of synovial fluid white blood cell count. Clin Orthop Related Res. 2011;469(1):34–40.
3. Della Valle CJ, Sporer SM, Jacobs JJ, Berger RA, Rosenberg AG, Paprosky WG. Preoperative testing for sepsis before revision total knee arthroplasty. J Arthroplasty. 2007;22(6 Suppl 2):90–3.
4. Christensen CP, Beair H, Della Valle CJ, Parvizi J, Schurko B, Jacobs C. The natural progression of synovial fluid white blood-cell counts and the percentage of polymorphonuclear cells after primary total knee arthroplasty: a multicenter study. J Bone Joint Surg Am. 2013;95(23):2081–7.

5. Della Valle CJ, Parvizi J, Bauer T, DiCesare P, Evans R, Segreti J, Spangehl M, Watters 3rd WC, Keith M, Turkelson C, Wies J, Sluka P, Hitchcock K. American Academy of Orthopaedic Surgeons clinical practice guideline on the diagnosis of periprosthetic joint infections of the hip and knee. J Bone Joint Surg Am. 2011;93(14):1355–7.

6. Parvizi J, Della Valle CJ. Culture negative periprosthetic joint infection. J Bone Joint Surg Am. 2014;96(5):430–6.

7. Tetreault MW, Wetters NG, Aggarwal VK, Moric M, Segreti J, Huddleston 3rd JI, Parvizi J, Della Valle CJ. Should draining wounds and sinuses associated with hip and knee arthroplasties be cultured? J Arthroplasty. 2013;28(8 Suppl):133–6.

8. Deirmengian C, Greenbaum J, Stern J, Braffman M, Lotke PA, Booth Jr RE, Lonner JH. Open debridement of acute gram-positive infections after total knee arthroplasty. Clin Orthop Relat Res. 2003;416:129–34.

9. Bradbury T, Fehring TK, Taunton M, Hanssen A, Azzam K, Parvizi J, Odum SM. The fate of acute methicillin-resistant Staphylococcus aureus periprosthetic knee infections treated by open debridement and retention of components. J Arthroplasty. 2009;24(6 Suppl):101–4.

10. Brown NM, Cipriano CA, Moric M, Sporer SM, Della Valle CJ. Dilute Betadine lavage before closure for the prevention of acute postoperative deep periprosthetic joint infection. J Arthroplasty. 2012;27(1):27–30.

11. Wyles CC, Taunton MJ, Jacobson SR, Tran NV, Sierra RJ, Trousdale RT. Intraoperative angiography provides objective assessment of skin perfusion in complex knee reconstruction. Clin Orthop Relat Res. 2014; [Epub ahead of print]. doi: 10.1007/s11999-014-3612-z.

Chapter 8
Periprosthetic Infection: Management of Late Acute Hematogenous Infection

Matthew Russo and Brian Evans

8.1 Case Presentation

The patient is a 54-year-old gentleman who underwent uncomplicated right total knee arthroplasty approximately 3 years prior who had no complaints with his knee until presentation. Approximately 3 days ago, he began to develop pain and swelling in the knee. He did not have any history of trauma or injury that may have resulted in pain. As the pain was increasing he presented to the emergency department for evaluation. Laboratory evaluation revealed the Erythrocyte sedimentation rate (ESR) was 29 mm/h and C-reactive protein (CRP) was 17.3 mg/L with a serum white blood cell count (WBC) of 12. Physical examination of the right knee revealed a moderate effusion and painful range of motion of 0–90°, minimal warmth but no erythema or drainage. He had good alignment without any varus or valgus instability. Aspiration of the joint revealed a synovial WBC count of 34,000 with a differential of 91 % neutrophils. Gram stain was positive for gram positive cocci with eventual

M. Russo, MD (✉) • B. Evans, MD
Department of Orthopedic Surgery, Medstar Georgetown
University Hospital, Washington, DC, USA
e-mail: matt.russo.md@gmail.com

© Springer International Publishing Switzerland 2015   91
B.D. Springer and B.M. Curtin (eds.), *Complex Primary
and Revision Total Knee Arthroplasty: A Clinical Casebook*,
DOI 10.1007/978-3-319-18350-3_8

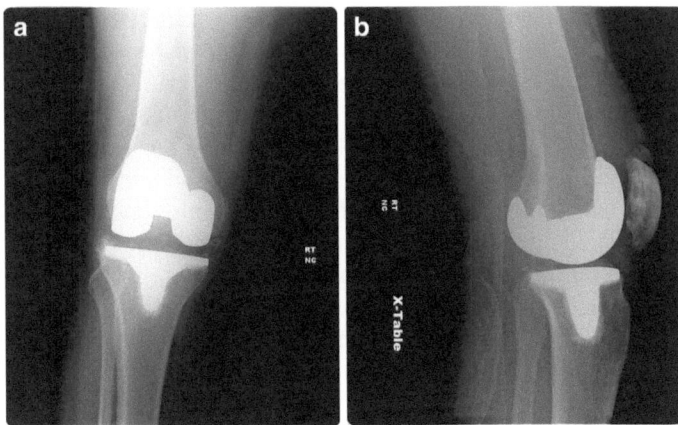

FIG. 8.1. AP (**a**) and lateral (**b**) X-rays on initial presentation demonstrating a stable right total knee arthroplasty with no evidence of loosening or mal-alignment.

growth of methicillin-sensitive staphylococcus aureus (MSSA). X-rays obtained on presentation showed no evidence of loosening or mal-alignment (Fig. 8.1). The patient recalls recent dental work performed a couple weeks ago. No prophylactic antibiotics were utilized at that time.

His past medical history is significant for protein-S deficiency for which he was on coumadin with an IVC filter in place, hypertension, depression, and coronary artery disease with history of a myocardial infarction. He had a contralateral total knee arthroplasty (TKA) performed approximately 4 years prior without complication. The initial implant used was a cemented posterior stabilized construct, with a rotating platform tibia and a resurfaced patella.

8.2   Management

Given the acute onset of symptoms and positive arthrocentesis, a diagnosis of acute late periprosthetic infection was made and the patient was taken the following day to the operating room for irrigation and debridement with polyethylene exchange. All infected-appearing tissue as well as the pseudo-membrane was removed. Betadine scrub brushes were utilized to scrub the femoral, tibial, and patellar components, which were noted to be well fixed with no signs of loosening. All previous ethibond sutures were removed and the wound was irrigated with 6 L of normal saline pulse lavage. A new polyethylene insert of the same size was implanted. A hemovac drain was placed prior to fascial closure with #1 prolene sutures. This was followed by 2-0 subcutaneous PDS suture. The skin was closed with staples.

Due to the patient's hypercoagulable state, he was placed on lovenox postoperatively and bridged back to coumadin. A peripherally inserted central catheter (PICC) was placed for 6 weeks of Cefepime in addition to oral Rifampin as recommended by an infectious disease consult obtained while in the hospital. His rehabilitation included range of motion exercises, full weight-bearing and gentle muscle strengthening similar to a primary total knee replacement.

Postoperatively, the patient did experience some pain relief but denied resolution of his pain. Approximately 2 months postoperatively (2 weeks after cessation of the IV antibiotic therapy), the patient returned with persistent right knee pain, erythema, and an effusion. Range of motion of the right knee was 0–105° with no evidence of instability. Repeat laboratory markers revealed an ESR of 25 mm/h, CRP of 21 mg/L, and a peripheral white blood cell count of 6. Aspiration was also performed at that time revealing 23,000 WBCs (differential of 92 % neutrophils) and cultures eventually growing MSSA.

The patient was taken back to the operating room after normalization of his INR for the first step of a two-stage exchange procedure for explant of the right knee arthroplasty and placement of a molded antibiotic-loaded knee spacer (Fig. 8.2) utilizing 3 g of tobramycin per cement package. The knee was closed in a similar fashion with hemovac drain in place. At the recommendation of infectious disease, the patient was given an additional 6 weeks of antibiotics consisting of daptomycin.

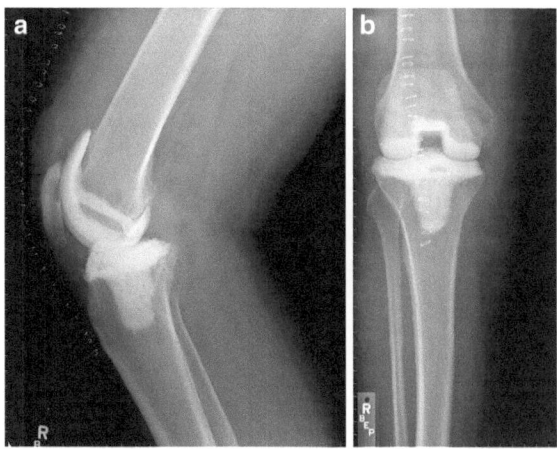

Fɪɢ. 8.2. Postoperative lateral (**a**) and AP (**b**) X-rays demonstrating insertion of antibiotic-loaded articulating spacer.

After explant, the patient was again bridged back to his coumadin with lovenox and began a physical therapy protocol in the attempt to maintain range of motion and to encourage weight-bearing. After completing his antibiotic course, his labs were again drawn demonstrating normalization of both ESR and CRP prior to reimplantation. The patient was replanted approximately 7 months later with a posterior stabilized revision construct consisting of hybrid diaphyseal engaging stems and porous metaphyseal sleeves on both the tibia and femur. Antibiotic cement was used in a limited fashion proximally under the tibial component and distally under the femoral component. Physical therapy following revision utilized the same protocol used following primary total knee replacement. Postoperatively, the patient recovered well and had no further complications with the knee.

8.3   Outcome

Most recent follow-up 5 years after reimplantation reveals the patient has healed his incision nicely with no complaints of pain, drainage, or instability of the knee. X-rays reveal

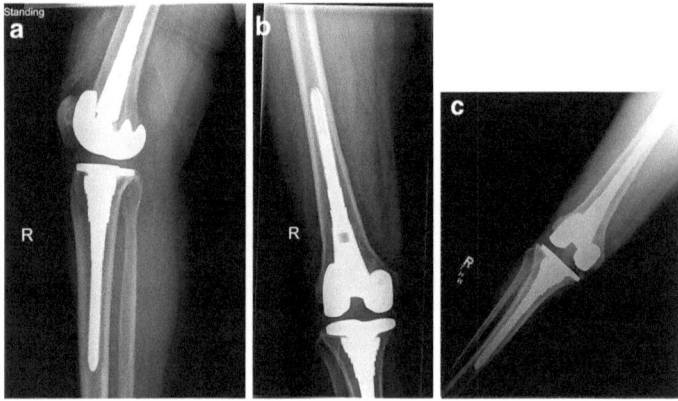

FIG. 8.3. Most recent lateral (**a**) and AP (**b, c**) X-rays after two-stage exchange arthroplasty.

well-fixed implants in good alignment (Fig. 8.3) with range of motion of approximately 5–110° actively and passively. He has been participating in physical therapy off and on and has returned to his preoperative level of activity without restriction.

8.4   Literature Review

8.4.1   Risk Factors

The typical presentation of a patient with late acute prosthetic knee infection is sudden onset of painful range of motion, swelling, and warmth in a previously well-functioning total knee implanted greater than 1 year [1]. There is growing evidence that the presence of diabetes with end-organ damage, heart disease, and pulmonary complications are important risk factors for the development of acute hematogenous infection [2]. Although no single comorbidity has shown to provide statistical significance for increased risk of infection, a total number of comorbidities greater than three as described by the Charlson comorbidity index has consistently been shown to be a significant risk factor in hematogenous infection [3].

In addition, Swan et al. [4] found that 88 % of late acute hematogenous prosthetic knee infections described some type of sentinel event prior to their diagnosis and presentation, with the most common being an open wound or skin infection. This finding has been supported also by Maderazo et al. [5] where similar organisms recovered from a distant skin source were also recovered in the infected joint.

A great amount of attention has also been given to the possible hematogenous spread of bacteria from the oral cavity after dental procedures. However, many authors discredit this belief due to the low incidence of streptococcal or oral pathogens ultimately grown from periprosthetic infections. In a 2010 case-control study by Berbari et al. [6], not only were dental procedures not a risk factor for subsequent periprosthetic infection but also patients who did take antibiotic prophylaxis did not decrease their rate of infection following a dental procedure. Although the connection between transient bacteremia and oral procedures appears to be well documented, there is no evidence that this bacteremia results in prosthetic joint infections.

8.4.2 Diagnosis

Diagnosis of periprosthetic infection in a previously well-functioning total knee is often a difficult task relying on risk stratification of patient risk factors as well as laboratory and imaging studies. First-line markers of infection include elevated inflammatory markers, both ESR and CRP. Although ESR and CRP serology labs have been recognized as helpful in establishing the diagnosis of prosthetic joint infection, there is no evidence to support the role of serum WBC [7]. Although nonspecific, advanced imaging may also be considered such as nuclear medicine bone scan or Positron Emission Tomography (PET) imaging, however bone scan studies without the use of labeled leukocytes have a limited role in the diagnosis of prosthetic joint infection. In the setting of elevated ESR >30 mm/h and CRP >10 mg/dL, with clinical suspicion for prosthetic joint infection, AAOS guidelines strongly recommend joint aspiration sent for gram stain, culture, and synovial fluid cell count with differential [8]. Furthermore, there is evidence that fluid samples directly injected into standard blood culture vials have the highest specificity, sensitivity, and accuracy (100, 92, and 94 %, respectively) compared with both culture swabs and tissue biopsy for identifying the infecting organism [9]. Synovial WBC >2,000/μL and neutrophil differential >70 % have historically been used as a rough measure for prosthetic joint infection, with recent Musculoskeletal Infection Society (MSIS) guidelines recommending a differential criteria of >1,100/μL for knees and >3,000/μL for hips [10]. It is important not to initiate any antibiotic treatment for presumed infection until after adequate aspiration of the joint has been performed and sent for culture.

8.4.3 Management

Once the diagnosis of acute hematogenous periprosthetic infection has been established in the setting of rapid onset of symptoms in a prior well-functioning joint, the mainstay of treatment remains early joint irrigation and debridement (I&D) with polyethylene exchange. The likelihood of this operation to successfully eradicate the infection has recently been called into question, with more favorable outcomes occurring in patients presenting early after the onset of symptoms, most notably before 2–4 weeks [11]. Azzam et al. [12] recently performed a retrospective review of 104 patients with periprosthetic knee and hip infections treated with initial I&D and component retention within 2 weeks of symptom onset, demonstrating a dismal 52 % success rate over 5 years as well as increased failure rate in patients with an elevated American Society of Anesthesiologists (ASA) score above 2 and presence of *staphylococcus aureus* (MSSA or MRSA). This study did however demonstrate a trend toward more successful eradication with I&D in patients presenting with late acute hematogenous infection compared with early postoperative infection, 60 % versus 48 %, respectively. Other studies have shown similar disappointing results, citing a 70 % recurrence rate after early I&D in patients with peri-prosthetic knee infection [13]. It also appears that this high failure rate is not completely dependent on the infecting organism, with a recent multicenter study demonstrating similar failure rates of early I&D with infection of either resistant or sensitive staphylococcal infections, at 76 and 72 %, respectively [14]. Despite its low success rate, early irrigation and debridement remains a common surgical option when compared to the more painful and morbid alternative of two-stage revision arthroplasty.

Postoperatively after early I&D, the patient is typically started on empiric intravenous antibiotics which are altered based on the results of the intraoperative cultures and sensitivities and continued for 6 weeks. The patient is then taken off all antibiotics with repeat blood tests performed 2–4 weeks after removal of antibiotics. In the setting of normal repeat inflammatory markers and absence of continued pain, the patient may be monitored in the clinic for an additional 6 months for evidence of any pain or swelling suggestive of ongoing infection.

If the patient returns with continued or worsening pain, repeat arthrocentesis and blood tests should be performed to confirm the diagnosis of persistent infection. As outlined in the case study provided above, management in this scenario often requires a two-stage revision arthroplasty for the proper eradication of infection.

8.5   Clinical Pearls/Pitfalls

- Late acute hematogenous infection is characterized by acute pain in a previously well-functioning prosthetic knee.
- Total number of comorbidities greater than three is a significant risk factor for hematogenous infection.

- Dental procedures are less likely to be considered sentinel infective events.
- Local skin infections specifically with staphylococcal species are highly correlated with increased rates of hematogenous infection.
- In the setting of elevated ESR >30 mm/h and CRP >10 mg/dL, aspiration should be performed. The fluid should be sent for cell count and differential and culture. Specimens for culture can be injected into blood culture vials for improved accuracy.
- Synovial WBC of >1,100/µL has been proposed as criteria for periprosthetic knee infections.
- Early irrigation and debridement with component retention is the mainstay of treatment, with improved outcomes and success rates associated with earlier treatment, specifically less than 2 weeks from the onset of symptoms.
- Failure to eradicate the infection with early irrigation and debridement necessitates component removal often in the form of a two-stage revision arthroplasty.

References

1. Pulido L, Ghanem E, Joshi A, Purtill JJ, Parvizi J. Periprosthetic joint infection: the incidence, timing, and predisposing factors. Clin Orthop Relat Res. 2008;466(7):1710–5.
2. Peersman G, Laskin R, Davis J, Peterson M. Infection in total knee replacement: a retrospective review of 6489 total knee replacements. Clin Orthop Relat Res. 2001;392:15–23.
3. Lai K, Bohm ER, Burnell C, Hedden DR. Presence of medical comorbidities in patients with infected primary hip or knee arthroplasties. J Arthroplasty. 2007;22:651–6.
4. Swan J, Dowsey M, Babazadeh S, Mandaleson A, Choong PF. Significance of sentinel infective events in haematogenous prosthetic knee infections. ANZ J Surg. 2011;81(1–2):40–5.
5. Maderazo EG, Judson S, Pasternak H. Late infections of total joint prostheses. A review and recommendations for prevention. Clin Orthop Relat Res. 1988;229:131–42.
6. Berbari EF, Osmon DR, Carr A, et al. Dental procedures as risk factors for prosthetic hip or knee infection: a hospital-based prospective case-control study. Clin Infect Dis. 2010;50(1):8–16.

7. Parvizi J, Della Valle CJ. AAOS Clinical Practice Guideline: diagnosis and treatment of periprosthetic joint infections of the hip and knee. J Am Acad Orthop Surg. 2010;18(12):771–2.
8. Della Valle C, Parvizi J, Bauer TW, DiCesare PE, Evans RP, Segreti J, Spangehl M, Watters 3rd WC, Keith M, Turkelson CM, Wies JL, Sluka P, Hitchcock K, American Academy of Orthopaedic Surgeons. American Academy of Orthopaedic Surgeons clinical practice guideline on: the diagnosis of periprosthetic joint infections of the hip and knee. J Bone Joint Surg Am. 2011;93(14):1355–7.
9. Levine BR, Evans BG. Use of blood culture vial specimens in intraoperative detection of infection. Clin Orthop Relat Res. 2001;382:222–31.
10. Parvizi J, Zmistowski B, Berbari EF, et al. New definition for periprosthetic joint infection: from the Workgroup of the Musculoskeletal Infection Society. Clin Orthop Relat Res. 2011;469(11):2992–4.
11. Marculescu CE, Berbari EF, Hanssen AD, et al. Outcome of prosthetic joint infections treated with debridement and retention of components. Clin Infect Dis. 2006;42:471.
12. Azzam KA, Seeley M, Ghanem E, Austin MS, Purtill JJ, Parvizi J. Irrigation and debridement in the management of prosthetic joint infection: traditional indications revisited. J Arthroplasty. 2010;25(7):1022–7.
13. Silva M, Tharani R, Schmalzried TP. Results of direct exchange or debridement of the infected total knee arthroplasty. Clin Orthop Relat Res. 2002;404:125–31.
14. Odum SM, Fehring TK, Lombardi AV, Zmistowski BM, Brown NM, Luna JT, Fehring KA, Hansen EN, Periprosthetic Infection Consortium. Irrigation and debridement for periprosthetic infections: does the organism matter? J Arthroplasty. 2011;26 (6 Suppl):114–8.

Chapter 9
Periprosthetic Infection: Management of Chronically Infected Total Knee Arthroplasty

Miguel M. Gomez, Jorge Manrique, and Javad Parvizi

9.1 Case Presentation

A 79-year-old male presented to our outpatient clinic with persistent pain and increasing effusion of the right knee, almost twice the size of the contralateral joint. The patient had an uneventful right total knee arthroplasty (TKA) 12 years ago. However, 4 years ago, he developed an acute hematogenous PJI caused by methicillin-sensitive *Staphylococcus aureus*. Subsequently, the patient underwent 8 procedures to control the infection, including multiple irrigation and debridements (I&D) and a two–stage exchange arthroplasty, with no improvement. The patient was then placed on suppressive oral therapy with doxycycline and referred to our institution.

Physical exam revealed an obese male with a body mass index (BMI) of 39 and hyperpigmentation around the incision, as well as warmth, tenderness, and painful range of motion. He had 30° of extension deficit and flexion was

M.M. Gomez, MD • J. Manrique, MD • J. Parvizi, MD, FRCS (✉)
The Rothman Institute at Thomas Jefferson University,
Philadelphia, PA, USA
e-mail: parvj@aol.com

© Springer International Publishing Switzerland 2015   101
B.D. Springer and B.M. Curtin (eds.), *Complex Primary and Revision Total Knee Arthroplasty: A Clinical Casebook*,
DOI 10.1007/978-3-319-18350-3_9

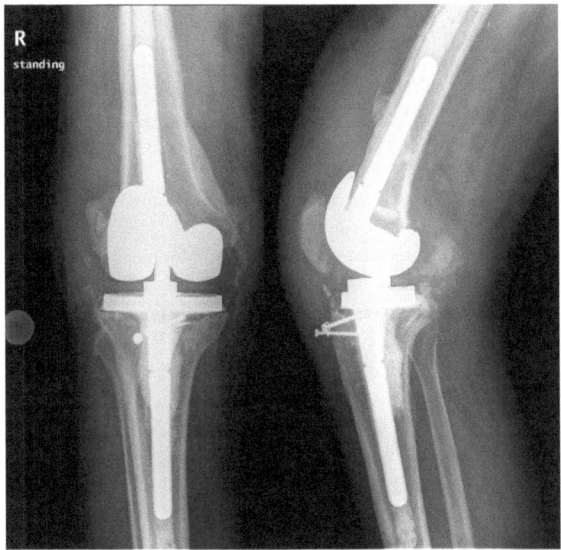

Fɪɢ. 9.1. Initial radiographs at first consultation.

limited to 90°. Radiographs showed a previously cemented long stem, with radiolucent areas around the cement-bone interface on the femoral side (Fig. 9.1). Serological markers demonstrated an erythrocyte sedimentation rate (ESR) of 78 mm/h and C-reactive protein (CRP) of 11.7 mg/dl.

The arthrocentesis was performed after the patient had been off of antibiotics for 3 weeks. Synovial fluid analysis revealed a synovial white cell count of 24,000 with 90 % polymorphonuclear cells. An extensor mechanism tear was suspected due to the lack of knee extension and a history of previous tibial tubercle osteotomy. Thus, a repeat two-stage exchange arthroplasty was performed.

9.2   Diagnosis/Assessment

The patient was diagnosed with a chronic right knee PJI. The diagnosis of PJI remains challenging due to confounding factors and lack of a gold standard test. The definition was first

TABLE 9.1. Periprosthetic joint infection (PJI) definition according to the International Joint Commission.

PJI is present when one of the major criteria exists or three out of five minor criteria exist	
Major criteria	1. Two positive periprosthetic cultures with phenotypically identical organisms
	2. A sinus tract communicating with the joint
Minor criteria	1. Elevated serum CRP **AND** ESR
	2. Elevated synovial fluid white blood cell count **OR** ++change on leukocyte esterase test strip
	3. Elevated synovial fluid polymorphonuclear neutrophil percentage
	4. >5 neutrophils per high power field in 5 high power fields (400×)
	5. A single positive culture

CRP C-reactive protein, *ESR* erythrocyte sedimentation rate
Modified from: Parvizi J, Gehrke T (2014) Definition of periprosthetic joint infection. J Arthroplasty 29:1331; used with permission

standardized by the Musculoskeletal Infection Society workgroup in 2011 [1]. This was later modified in 2013 by the International Consensus Meeting (ICM) on PJI [2]; the definition consisted of two major criteria and five minor criteria that must be present for diagnosis (Table 9.1). PJI is confirmed when one major or three minor criteria are met.

The American Academy of Orthopedic Surgeons (AAOS) has developed a clinical guideline to successfully diagnose PJI [3]. The guideline acts as a flowchart as opposed to a fixed protocol. The initial step is risk stratification of individuals to determine whether or not they are at high or low risk of developing PJI. In this particular case, the patient was considered to be at higher risk because he exhibited two symptoms related to PJI: pain and stiffness [3]. Along with increased temperature, the knee was swollen. A positive history of PJI and obesity are risk factors that are supported in the literature [4, 5]. Another important aspect of this case is early implant loosening (<5 years), which has been associated with a positive likelihood ratio (LR) of infection of 2.1 (1.36, 3.25; 95 % confidence interval [CI]) and a negative LR of 0.53 (0.29, 0.96; 95 % CI).

The next step involved investigating ESR and CRP. The ICM thresholds for chronic infections are stated [3] as >30 mm/h and >10 mg/L for ESR and CRP, respectively. Recently a positive leukocyte esterase test was added as a minor criterion, according to the ICM [2]. If the inflammatory markers are negative, the probability of infection is unlikely (negative LR: 0.0–0.06) and infection can be ruled out. However, if both are positive (positive LR: 4.3–12.1), a conclusive diagnosis of infection is not established and warrants further workup due to many variables and diseases that can skew the final result of the inflammatory markers. Positivity of the markers stratifies the patient into the high-risk group for infection and means that the patient needs further investigation.

If positive inflammatory markers are identified, a synovial fluid sample should be obtained. The superolateral approach is preferred to obtain synovial fluid from the knee; the use of contrast or local anesthetic should be avoided, since their antimicrobial activity may lead to a false negative [6].

The patient should be taken off antibiotic therapy for at least 2 weeks prior to obtaining intra-articular cultures [7]. The fluid should be tested for synovial white cells and polymorphonuclear cells, with a threshold for chronic PJI of >3,000 (cells/μ[mu]l) and >80 %, respectively, for chronic infections [3].

9.3   Management

The patient underwent the first stage of treatment, which consisted of removing all the prosthetic components, bone cement, and foreign material; and an extended synovectomy and implantation of a dynamic spacer with antibiotic-loaded bone cement. The extensor mechanism was intact and the tibial tubercle osteotomy had consolidated. Two cultures were positive for *Staphylococcus coagulase negative* and the infectious disease team was consulted, recommending intravenous vancomycin for 6 weeks. The patient was seen by a physical therapist, an occupational therapist, and a social

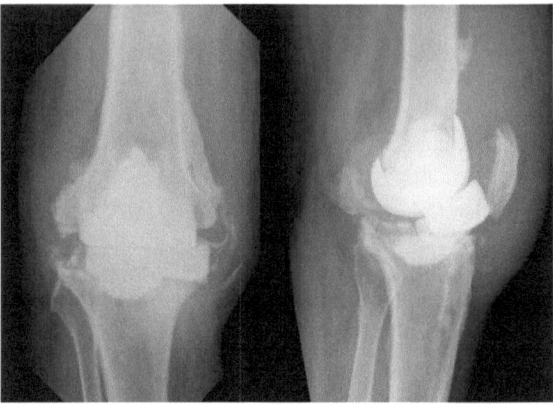

FIG. 9.2. AP and lateral view of the initial dynamic spacer showing the anterior shift of the tibial component.

worker, postoperatively. At discharge, he was able to toe-touch weight bear and was placed in a hinged brace that restricted range of motion from 0° up to 60°.

After a course of antibiotics, the knee remained swollen and painful during gait. Inflammatory markers remained above normal. Throughout this time the patient suffered from multiple urinary tract infections, which could have affected the results of the inflammatory markers. The synovial fluid cell count decreased compared to initial values but remained abnormal. On plain films, it was noted that the tibial component had failed and shifted anteriorly (Fig. 9.2). Three months after the first stage of the procedure, there was a high suspicion of persistent infection, and the patient was scheduled to undergo a spacer exchange and repeat I&D.

A new dynamic spacer was implanted and a thorough synovectomy was performed with removal of all foreign material. Clinically, the appearance of the knee was benign. Cultures taken during the spacer exchange procedure were all negative. With intraoperative findings, negative cultures, and a clinical improvement during the follow up period, the

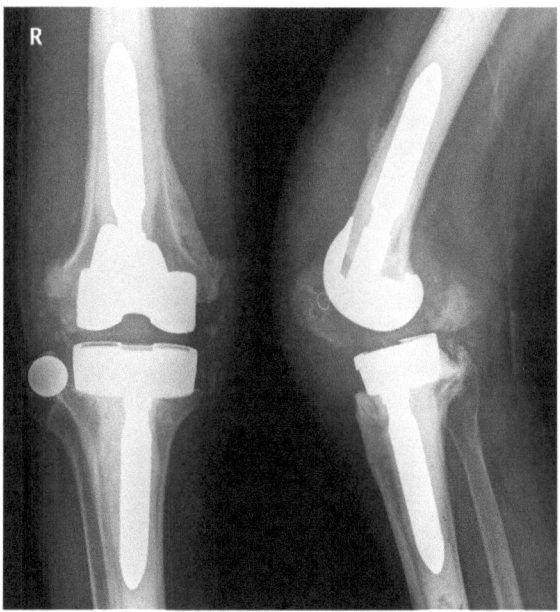

FIG. 9.3. Radiographs showing the prosthesis used after the second reimplantation.

patient was scheduled for reimplantation at 5 weeks after the spacer exchange.

Reimplantation occurred without any complications (Fig. 9.3). At the time of reimplantation, two cultures were positive for *Candida ssp*. Given these findings, the infectious disease team recommended placing the patient on long-term suppressive therapy, including antibiotics and antifungal therapy. Within the first year of reimplantation, the patient presented with mild effusion and minimal pain, tolerating gait without external support. Two years after reimplantation, pain and swelling increased and the patient's function diminished. The inflammatory markers were noted to increase and a new synovial aspiration was demonstrated to be above the threshold cell count. The patient was considered to benefit from a new I&D, although intraoperatively the decision was

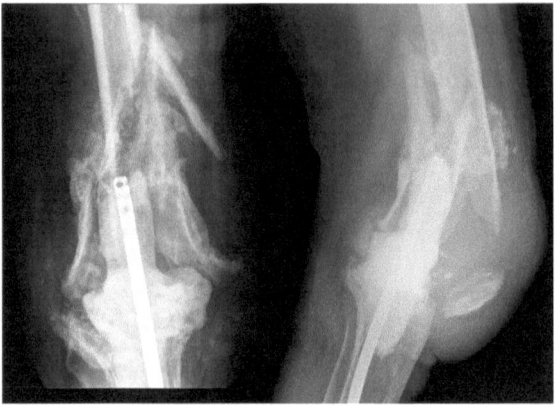

FIG. 9.4. Final radiographs and result of a static retained spacer and femoral shaft fracture with advanced healing.

made to perform a two-stage exchange arthroplasty. At this time a static spacer that contained antibiotic and antifungal loaded cement bone was chosen. In follow-up, the patient sustained a diaphyseal peri-spacer femoral fracture (Fig. 9.4). The fracture was managed nonoperatively due to lack of pain. At this point the patient was not considered a suitable candidate for reconstruction; he was placed on lifelong antibiotic suppression therapy and was able to walk with the use of external support and a brace.

9.4 Outcome

The two-stage exchange is the preferred treatment method to eradicate chronic PJI in patients in North America [8]. The procedure includes removal of all prosthetic components and foreign material, followed by I&D and implantation of an antibiotic-load bone cement spacer. A course of antibiotics, ranging from 6 to 12 weeks, follows this procedure. When infection is considered controlled, antibiotic treatment is withdrawn for a minimum of 2 weeks to serve as a proxy of infection control followed by a second stage with definitive reimplantation. The two-stage exchange offers the highest and most consistent rate of infection eradication compared with other treatment modalities, with a reported overall success rate ranging from 82 to 100 % [9].

However, this treatment option has complications, which are usually worse than the infection itself. The incidence of recurrent or persistent infection after a two-stage procedure for the knee ranges from 9 to 33 %. Predictors of failure have been identified for two-stage exchange, including culture negativity in the first stage, gram negative organism infection, methicillin-resistant organism infection, and increased reimplantation operative time [10].

The patient underwent a spacer exchange during the treatment course due to persistence of the infection and displacement of the components. Spacers provide local release of antibiotics, an increase of joint stability, prevention of soft tissue contractures, and potentially easier reimplantation [11]. The decision to use dynamic spacers took into account adequate bone stock and good quality soft tissues. Dynamic spacers are associated with a greater range of motion (ROM) after the second stage, with an average ROM of 101° for dynamic spacers compared to 91° for static spacers. The reinfection rate appears to be unaffected by the type of spacer used [12]. However, problems related to the spacer are not infrequent, accounting for up to 57 % of the complications. Of these, 13 % are major problems including fractures and dislocation of the knee [13].

At the time of reimplantation, the patient had two cultures positive for *Candida ssp,* contributing to a worse outcome. Periprosthetic fungal infection is a rare but devastating complication, and its management is a challenge. There is no agreement in the literature regarding the ideal treatment option. The ICM for PJI in 2013 attempted to summarize the available information regarding fungal infection treatment. According to the ICM recommendations, fungi infection should be considered if a fungal pathogen is isolated from periprosthetic tissue cultures or joint aspiration in a patient who has signs and symptoms of PJI and not assumed to be a contaminant. Host factors predisposing a patient to fungal PJI are immunosuppression, malignancy, antineoplastic therapy, drug abuse, prolonged use of antibiotics, prolonged use of indwelling catheters, diabetes mellitus, malnutrition, rheumatoid arthritis, history of multiple abdominal surgeries, severe burns, tuberculosis, and prior bacterial infection of the prosthesis.

Two-stage exchange arthroplasty is the recommended treatment for fungal PJI. However, the success rate is lower than that of bacterial cases, with only 50 % of patients not requiring further surgical intervention for infection [12]. The spacer cement is usually loaded with both antibacterial and antifungal agents. The most frequent agents are liposomal amphotericin B and voriconazole, the latter of which affects the cement's mechanical strength [14]. Systemic antifungal treatment should be initiated after the first stage and continued for at least 6 weeks. To monitor fungal PJI cases, a serial CRP and ESR should be taken. The timing to reimplantation is based on clinical judgment and normalization of inflammatory values. There is no support for continuing antifungal agents after reimplantation [14].

After a failed two-stage reimplantation, a second two-stage procedure may be performed, taking into account the virulence of the infecting organism, underlying medical conditions, bone stock, soft tissue integrity, and patient desires. After a repeat procedure is performed, the rate of infection control reaches 77 %, but 64 % of these cases required long-term antibiotic or antifungal suppression for at least 6 months [15]. We made three attempts to treat PJI in our patient without success, and we made the decision to retain the spacer along with long-term suppressive antibiotic therapy. In patients in whom unplanned spacer retention occurs, return to daily function occurs in 60 % of cases, with a mean follow up of 6 years after insertion [16]. The patient in our case study had lower than expected function, but an attempt to pursue reconstruction could have resulted in a worse outcome, such as loss of the extremity.

9.5   Clinical Pearls/Pitfalls

- The use of the current definition of PJI by ICM is advised.
- Clinical judgment must prevail and every case must be considered individually. However, it is strongly recommended to follow the flowchart proposed by the AAOS in order to make an accurate diagnosis of PJI.
- Currently available diagnostic tests are highly sensitive and less specific, leading to a high rate of false positive cases.
- Screening and stratifying risk factors must be performed to adequately assess the patient.
- Treatment should be carried out by an adult joint reconstruction surgeon.
- Multidisciplinary assessment of the infected patient must be carried out.
- Two-stage exchange reimplantation is the preferred treatment for PJI, showing a high success rate.
- A second two-stage exchange arthroplasty is a suitable option after failure of the initial treatment.
- PJI caused by fungal organisms poses a challenge for management and is associated with bad outcomes.
- The use of a retained spacer should only be considered once other options have been exhausted, and the benefit outweighs the risk.
- Suppression antibiotic therapy is limited to patients without reconstruction options.
- The patient must always be advised of the potential complications after a primary TKA.

References

1. Parvizi J, Zmistowski B, Berbari EF, Bauer TW, Springer BD, Della Valle CJ, Garvin KL, Mont MA, Wongworawat MD, Zalavras CG. New definition for periprosthetic joint infection: from the Workgroup of the Musculoskeletal Infection Society. Clin Orthop Relat Res. 2011;469:2992–4.

2. Parvizi J, Gehrke T. Definition of periprosthetic joint infection. J Arthroplasty. 2014;29:1331.
3. Della Valle C, Parvizi J, Bauer TW, et al. American Academy of Orthopaedic Surgeons clinical practice guideline on: the diagnosis of periprosthetic joint infections of the hip and knee. J Bone Joint Surg Am. 2011;93:1355–7.
4. Jämsen E, Huhtala H, Puolakka T, Moilanen T. Risk factors for infection after knee arthroplasty. A register-based analysis of 43,149 cases. J Bone Joint Surg Am. 2009;91:38–47.
5. Dowsey MM, Choong PFM. Obese diabetic patients are at substantial risk for deep infection after primary TKA. Clin Orthop Relat Res. 2009;467:1577–81.
6. Schmidt RM, Rosenkranz HS. Antimicrobial activity of local anesthetics: lidocaine and procaine. J Infect Dis. 1970;121: 597–607.
7. Osmon DR, Berbari EF, Berendt AR, Lew D, Zimmerli W, Steckelberg JM, Rao N, Hanssen A, Wilson WR. Executive summary: diagnosis and management of prosthetic joint infection: clinical practice guidelines by the Infectious Diseases Society of America. Clin Infect Dis. 2013;56:1–10.
8. Parvizi J, Zmistowski B, Adeli B. Periprosthetic joint infection: treatment options. Orthopedics. 2010;33:659.
9. Jämsen E, Stogiannidis I, Malmivaara A, Pajamäki J, Puolakka T, Konttinen YT. Outcome of prosthesis exchange for infected knee arthroplasty: the effect of treatment approach. Acta Orthop. 2009;80:67–77.
10. Mortazavi SMJ, Vegari D, Ho A, Zmistowski B, Parvizi J. Two-stage exchange arthroplasty for infected total knee arthroplasty: predictors of failure. Clin Orthop Relat Res. 2011;469:3049–54.
11. Munro JT, Garbuz DS, Masri BA, Duncan CP. Articulating antibiotic impregnated spacers in two-stage revision of infected total knee arthroplasty. J Bone Joint Surg Br. 2012;94:123–5.
12. Voleti PB, Baldwin KD, Lee G-C. Use of static or articulating spacers for infection following total knee arthroplasty: a systematic literature review. J Bone Joint Surg Am. 2013;95:1594–9.
13. Struelens B, Claes S, Bellemans J. Spacer-related problems in two-stage revision knee arthroplasty. Acta Orthop Belg. 2013; 79:422–6.
14. Gebauer M, Frommelt L, Achan P, et al. Management of fungal or atypical periprosthetic joint infections. J Arthroplasty. 2014; 29:112–4.

15. Azzam K, McHale K, Austin M, Purtill JJ, Parvizi J. Outcome of a second two-stage reimplantation for periprosthetic knee infection. Clin Orthop Relat Res. 2009;467:1706–14.
16. Choi H-R, Freiberg AA, Malchau H, Rubash HE, Kwon Y-M. The fate of unplanned retention of prosthetic articulating spacers for infected total hip and total knee arthroplasty. J Arthroplasty. 2014;29:690–3.

Chapter 10
Revision Total Knee Arthroplasty: Management of Deficient Extensor Mechanism

Clint Wooten and Bryan D. Springer

10.1   Case Presentation

A 60-year-old morbidly obese female presented to the office 5 years out from an uncomplicated left total knee arthroplasty. One year prior she sustained a mechanical fall and suffered a displaced patella fracture with disruption of her extensor mechanism. Attempts were made to primarily repair the patella fracture with suture anchors. The repair failed and the patient was left with a severe extensor lag of 70° and the inability to fully straighten the leg. She was unable to ambulate without the use of a hinged brace locked in extension and was unable to perform a straight leg raise. Radiographs shown in Fig. 10.1 reveal failed fixation of the patella fracture with superior displacement of the patella fragment and disruption of the extensor mechanism.

Because of the patients' severe disability, the decision was made to proceed to surgery for extensor mechanism reconstruction. Because previous attempts at primary repair had

C. Wooten, MD • B.D. Springer, MD (✉)
OrthoCarolina Hip and Knee Center, Charlotte, NC, USA
e-mail: bryan.springer@orthocarolina.com

© Springer International Publishing Switzerland 2015   113
B.D. Springer and B.M. Curtin (eds.), *Complex Primary and Revision Total Knee Arthroplasty: A Clinical Casebook*,
DOI 10.1007/978-3-319-18350-3_10

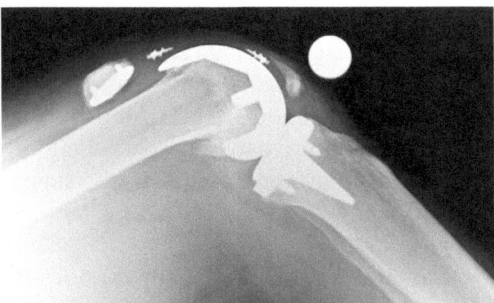

Fig. 10.1. Lateral radiographs demonstrating disruption of the extensor mechanism through a failed attempt at fixation of a displaced patella fracture.

failed, there were concerns about the patient's native host tissue. The decision was made to use a whole extensor mechanism allograft to reconstruct the extensor mechanism.

10.2   Incidence of Extensor Mechanism Disruption

Extensor mechanism (EM) disruption is an uncommon complication following total knee arthroplasty. Disruption can occur at the level of the patellar tendon, the patella with a concomitant fracture, or the quadriceps tendon. The overall incidence of extensor mechanism disruption has been reported between 1.1 and 6.6 % [1]. Risk factors include multiply operated knees, systemic conditions such as renal disease, diabetes, systemic steroid use, rheumatoid arthritis, and obesity [2, 3]. Iatrogenic injury at the time of surgery is unfortunately a common cause. Iatrogenic injury stems from failure to protect the extensor mechanism, especially in a patient with a stiff knee where exposure may be difficult and common particularly in revision surgery.

Quadriceps tendon rupture is the least common site of disruption. Dobbs et al. identified 24 of 23,800 TKA patients (0.1 %) from the Mayo Clinic with a partial or complete quadriceps tendon rupture [4]. Several risk factors exist. Aggressive resection of the patella can compromise the insertion of the quadriceps. Vascular injury may be a risk factor as well. In the previous referenced study, all three patients with quadriceps tendon rupture had undergone a lateral retinacular release [4]. This may cause injury to the superior lateral genicular artery and place the tendon at heightened risk for rupture.

Patellar fractures after TKA usually do not interrupt the extensor mechanism. Vertical fractures can typically be treated without surgery unless there is component loosening. More recently, the incidence of all patellar fractures has ranged from 0.3 to 5.4 % [5]. A study from Mayo clinic identified 85 fractures after 12,464 TKAs (0.68 %) of which only 12 were associated with extensor mechanism rupture [6]. Sinha et al. discussed three major risk factors that statistically increased the risk of patella fracture: resurfacing or over-resection of the patella, implant malalignment, or compromise of the patellar blood supply via lateral retinacular release [5]. All efforts should be made to prevent these risk factors.

Patellar tendon rupture or avulsion has been reported in as many as 2.5 % of patients with TKA [2]. Risk factors include difficult exposure in the setting of revision surgery, previous high tibial osteotomy, previous patellar realignment surgery, or systemic disease. Several techniques to gain exposure have been recommended to protect the patellar tendon during surgery including resection of intra-articular scar, quadriceps snip, and tibial tubercle osteotomy.

10.3   Diagnosis/Evaluation

In this case presentation, the disruption of the extensor mechanism occurred at the level of the patella following a traumatic fall. Primary repair of the patella and/or extensor mechanism in the setting of total knee arthroplasty often leads to suboptimal results and is associated with high rates of failure as discussed in the outcomes section below. In this case, attempts to repair the patella fracture with suture anchors led to suboptimal fixation and failure requiring extensor mechanism reconstruction.

When assessing a patient with possible extensor mechanism disruption, it is important to perform a thorough history and physical exam. While often times the extensor deficiency is obvious, there are several critical issues that should be addressed that have a key role in the etiology and ultimately the outcome of the extensor mechanism reconstruction. These elements include the chronicity of the injury, previous surgeries, or complications from previous surgery, particularly if they involved the extensor mechanism. The patient's current health and functional status is also important. Every patient should be questioned and evaluated about signs and symptoms of infection.

The physical exam should focus on the function of the extensor mechanism as well as the status of the soft tissue envelope. Inability to perform active knee extension or inability to do a straight leg raise indicates dysfunction of the extensor mechanism. A palpable defect in the patellar tendon or quadriceps may be felt on exam, along with the presence of a "high riding" patella if the patella tendon is disrupted. Often the patient may present with a large effusion in the knee that is subcutaneous from extravasation of the joint fluid from the disrupted extensor mechanism. In addition to infection, instability or component mal-rotation may be the cause for extensor mechanism disruption and must be addressed prior to the reconstruction. Failure to correct the errors at the time of surgery will lead to high failure rates of the reconstruction and the surgeon must be prepared to revise all necessary components at the time of extensor mechanism reconstruction as needed.

Plain radiographs are often all that is needed to assist in the diagnosis. The lateral radiograph may show patella alta, or a high riding patella as in this case (Fig. 10.1). Both the femoral and tibial components should be evaluated for loosening, osteolysis, and malposition.

CT scan and MRI are useful adjuncts in the diagnosis of patellar tendon ruptures if it is not readily evident on physical exam and plain radiographs. Recent advances in metal artifact reduction sequences have allowed better characterization of the remaining host tissue to assist in surgical decision making. CT scan can be used to determine femoral or tibial mal-rotation that may require revision at the time of surgery.

The surgeon also needs to assess the patient's candidacy for a relatively lengthy rehabilitation process that will require strict postoperative protocols. Contraindications to extensor mechanism reconstruction would include active periprosthetic infection and medical comorbidities precluding surgical intervention as well as a patient who is unwilling or unable to comply with postoperative protocols.

10.4 Management and Treatment Options

10.4.1 Nonoperative

Patients that are poor reconstruction candidates may be better treated with bracing or arthrodesis. Nonoperative treatment will require full dependency on gait aids and/or the use of knee braces. A brace that locks into extension (drop lock brace) when the patient is ambulating and have a drop-down lever to unlock the brace so that when they sit the knee is able to flex typically provides the best support. Despite this treatment, these patients typically remain functionally dependent on assistive devices.

10.4.2 Primary Repair

Primary repair of the extensor mechanism has largely been abandoned secondary to poor outcomes [7]. Despite successful results with primary repair in the native knee, similar treatment in the TKA patient has not seen similar success and is associated with high rates of complications with poor outcomes. Two studies looked at 23 combined patients and found 21 patients that were clinical failures with most common cause being rerupture [4,7]. These poor results prompted interest in alternative techniques for reconstruction.

10.4.3   Allograft Reconstruction

Extensor mechanism reconstruction with allograft has long been the mainstay of treatment and has demonstrated significantly better outcomes than primary repair. Allograft reconstruction was first reported by Emerson and colleagues in 1990 [8]. Several studies of this and other allograft reconstruction techniques have helped establish important surgical principles with improved outcomes.

Allograft tissue has the advantages of providing good tissue to augment the poor host tissue. Fresh frozen allografts have better strength and less immunogenic potential than freeze-dried grafts. There are concerns, however, about disease transmission with the use of allograft tissue. The two most commonly described allograft techniques include the use of either a (1) whole extensor mechanism allograft or (2) Achilles tendon allograft. These techniques are applicable to a wide range of extensor mechanism disruptions. Achilles tendon is best used when the patella and patellar tendon are intact. More recently, newer techniques utilizing synthetic grafts have been reported and have the advantage of ease of availability and lower cost [9].

10.4.4   Surgical Technique for Whole Extensor Mechanism Allograft Reconstruction

The case presented in this chapter was reconstructed with a whole extensor mechanism allograft that consists of a tibial bone block, patella tendon, patella, and quadriceps tendon. The following steps outline the surgical technique.

10.4.4.1   Presurgical Inspection of the Allograft

It is imperative for the surgeon to directly inspect the allograft prior to surgery to ensure that the appropriate side has been obtained (e.g., left vs. right) and that there is at least 5 cm of tibial bone present to allow for distal fixation and 5 cm of quadriceps tendon proximally. The use of a whole proximal tibial allograft allows the surgeon to intraoperatively customize the size of the tibial bone block.

10.4.4.2   Surgical Exposure

The patient is positioned supine on the operating room table. Depending on the length of the leg and the need for a longer incision, a nonsterile or sterile tourniquet can be utilized. Prior incisions should be utilized when possible. The previous extensor mechanism can be split longitudinally and dissected off the bone to expose the proximal tibia. The previous patella can be shelled out of the extensor mechanism and removed.

10.4.4.3   Allograft Preparation

It is helpful to have a second surgical team prepare the allograft on the back table. The allograft tibial bone block should be in general 5 cm in length, 2 cm in depth, and 2 cm in width to allow for solid fixation into the host tibia (Fig. 10.2). A dovetail should be created in the proximal portion of the tibial allograft to allow it to be slotted into the native host tibia. Generally this is done in a distal anterior to proximal posterior direction at approximately a 30–45° angle (Fig. 10.3). It is not necessary or recommended to resurface the allograft patella.

10.4.4.4   Preparation of the Host Tibia

The proximal portion of the trough in the host tibia should start no less than 15 mm below the host tibial bone to prevent graft escape or proximal fracture. The trough can be outlined

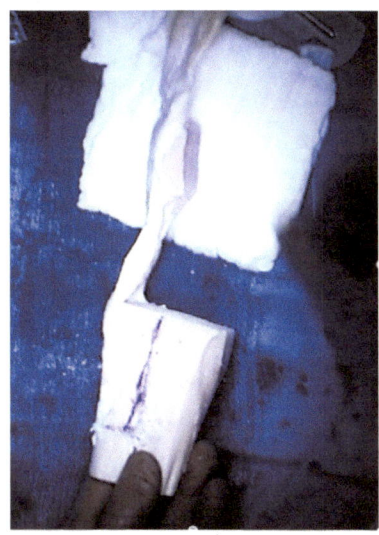

FIG. 10.2. The whole proximal tibial allograft allows for customization of the allograft tibial bone block. The bone block should, if possible, be 5 cm in length, 2 cm in width, and 2 cm in depth.

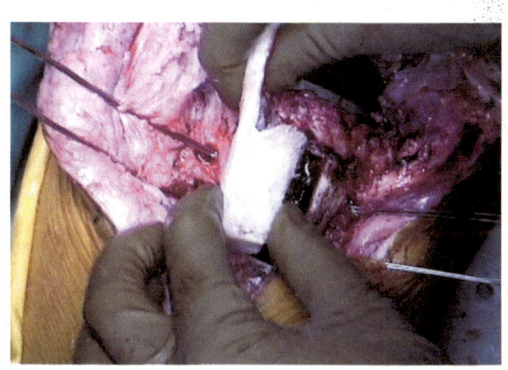

FIG. 10.3. A dovetail is created in the bone block from distal anterior to proximal posterior. This allows the allograft to be slotted into the native tibia for extra stability.

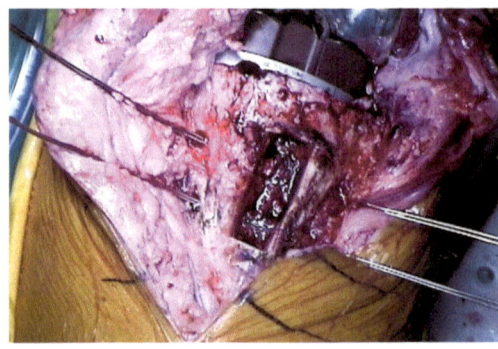

Fɪɢ. 10.4. Two to three wires are placed posterior to the tibial slot to allow for fixation of the allograft tibial bone.

with a marking pen and the dimensions should be made slightly less than that of the allograft bone block to allow for a secure press-fit. Two to three 16 or 18 gauge wires can be placed through drill holes in the tibia to allow for secure fixation (Fig. 10.4). If a stemmed component is to be used, the trial component should be in place when the trough is made to ensure that the wires can be safely passed without interfering with the position of the stemmed component. Once the trough has been prepared, the allograft tissue is dovetailed into the trough and gently tapped into place. The wires are then sequentially tightened, twisted, and bent laterally to allow for appropriate soft tissue coverage (Fig. 10.5).

10.4.4.5 Preparation of Proximal Portion of Allograft and Host Quadriceps Tendon

The proximal portion of the allograft is then secured on both sides with heavy nonabsorbable suture placed in a running, locking fashion along the medial and lateral aspects of the tendon, creating four free strands of suture proximally (Fig. 10.6). The knee is then brought into full extension. The extensor mechanism allograft tissue is tensioned by an assistant proximally. Sutures or clamps can be used to secure the host quadriceps mechanism and these are pulled distally over

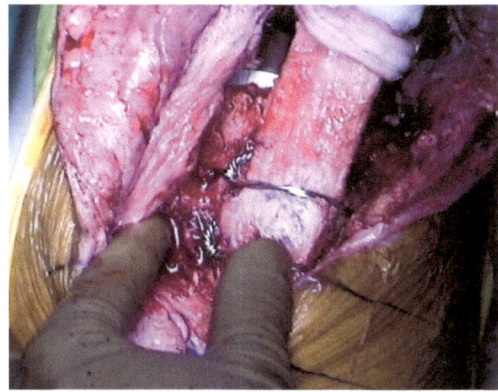

FIG. 10.5. The wires are tightened for fixation of the allograft to the host bone.

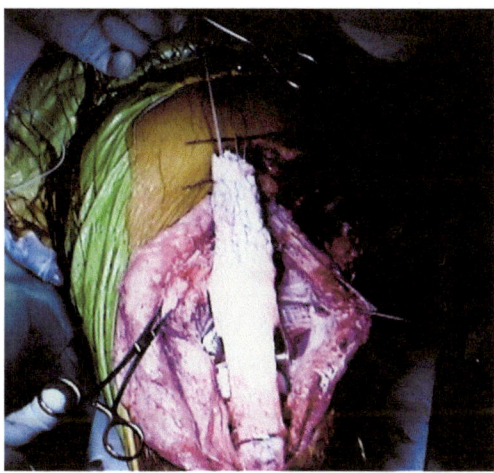

FIG. 10.6. The proximal portion of the allograft tendon is sutured with heavy nonabsorbable suture in a running locking fashion.

the top of the allograft quadriceps tendon. The host quadriceps is then sewn over the top of the allograft in a "pants-over-vest" technique, using nonabsorbable suture (Fig. 10.7). It is extremely important at this step that maximal tension is

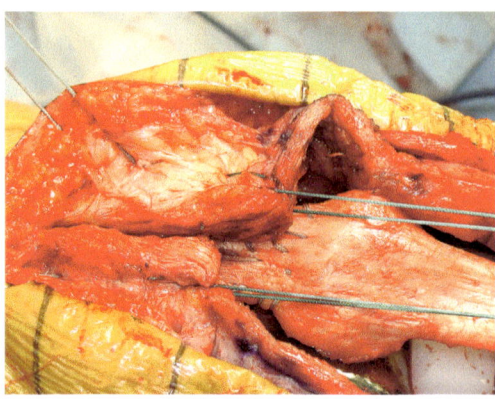

Fig. 10.7. The allograft is then pulled proximally and the native host quadriceps tendon is pulled distally and sutured together under maximum tension in full extension.

kept on the allograft and host tissue while the allograft is being sewn into place. Additionally, one must not at anytime flex the knee to test the stability of the graft. It must remain in full extension at all times. Closure allows for the entire allograft to be covered with native host tissue (Fig. 10.8).

10.4.4.6 Postoperative Management

Appropriate postoperative management requires strict adherence to protocol and is essential to the success of extensor mechanism reconstruction. Patients are placed in a rigid long leg cast postoperatively and allowed to be partial weight bearing with an assistive device. The cast should remain in place for a minimum of 6–8 weeks and changed when necessary. At 4–6 weeks the patient may begin doing quadricep sets and assistive straight leg raises in the cast.

When the cast is removed, the patient should be placed in a hinged knee brace. The patient may then begin to weight bear as tolerated if the radiographs show incorporation of the allograft bone block. In addition, quad sets and straight leg raises are continued. The hinged knee brace is unlocked to

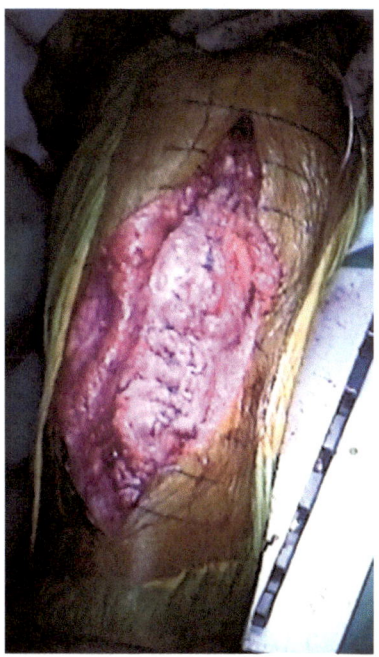

Fig. 10.8. Closure allows for native tissue to completely cover the allograft extensor mechanism.

allow 0–30° of flexion and flexion is increased by 20–30° every 2–3 weeks. Patients should avoid passive flexion of the knee by a therapist to prevent stretching of the graft. Flexion should be done against gravity or actively by the patient. Active and active assisted extension is allowed. Once the patient reaches 90° of flexion (generally 6–8 weeks after cast removal), the brace can be removed and gradual increase in flexion is allowed.

10.5   Outcome

The patient tolerated the surgical procedure well. She was placed on 6 weeks of chemical thromboprophylaxis while immobilized in the cast. She was compliant with the postoperative rehabilitation protocols and at 6 months from surgery was ambulating without the need of any assistive devices. She had active full extension with no apparent flexion lag and flexion to 115°.

10.6   Literature Review

There is a relative paucity of clinical literature on extensor mechanism reconstruction, owing to its relative rarity as a complication as well as the variety of techniques described. Reconstruction with an allograft has the most supporting literature, but still suffers from low patient numbers and some early variation in technique that led to poor outcomes. Leopold et al. (1999) reported their results of whole extensor mechanism allografts in seven patients [10]. At an average clinical follow-up of 30 months, all seven were deemed clinical failures as each had extensor lags of at least 30° and most required ambulatory aids.

In 1999, Nazarian and Booth described the maximal tensioning of the allograft in full extension [11]. This technical change has led to improvement in success and functional outcomes of this procedure. At an average follow-up of 3.6 years, 36 patients had an average extensor lag of 13° and 23 patients had active full extension. Burnett compared the results of these two techniques [12]. In the nontensioned group, the average extensor lag was 59° and all patients were considered clinical failures. In the group that included the allograft tensioned in extension, the average extensor lag was 4.3° and all patients had improvement in Knee Society scores. These two studies emphasize the important technical aspect of placing and keeping maximal tension on the graft during the repair and in the postoperative period.

Brown and Hanssen have reported on a series of 13 patients that underwent reconstruction of a ruptured patellar tendon with the use of a synthetic mesh [9]. The surgical technique is well described in this article. There were three cases of graft failure and one case of failure for recurrent sepsis.

The remaining nine patients had an average extensor lag of 2.8°. The cost of the synthetic mesh at the author's institution was $122.00 compared to $4,437.45 for a whole extensor mechanism allograft. While the result of this technique is early, the use of synthetic mesh for reconstruction of extensor mechanism dysfunction may be a cost-effective means for reconstruction compared to the use of allograft tissue.

10.7   Clinical Pearls/Pitfalls

- Extensor mechanism disruption is an infrequent but devastating complication following total knee arthroplasty.
- Preventive efforts through identification of at-risk patients and meticulous surgical technique are essential to minimize risk of disruption of the extensor mechanism.
- Allograft extensor mechanism reconstruction is the most published and studied technique.
- Tensioning of the allograft in full extension is of critical importance for the success of the surgical technique.
- Patellar resurfacing of the allograft patella is unnecessary.
- Postoperative protocol is critical. Immobilizing the leg in extension for 6–8 weeks is recommended before the introduction of gradual range of motion.

References

1. Aracil J, Salom M, Aroca JE, Torro V, Lopez-Quiles D. Extensor apparatus reconstruction with Leeds-Keio ligament in total knee arthroplasty. J Arthroplasty. 1999;14(2):204–8.
2. Lynch AF, Rorabeck CH, Bourne RB. Extensor mechanism complications following total knee arthroplasty. J Arthroplasty. 1987;2(2):135–40.
3. Springer BD, Della Valle CJ. Extensor mechanism allograft reconstruction after total knee arthroplasty. J Arthroplasty. 2008; 23(7 Suppl):35–8.
4. Dobbs RE, Hanssen AD, Lewallen DG, Pagnano MW. Quadriceps tendon rupture after total knee arthroplasty. Prevalence, complications, and outcomes. J Bone Joint Surg. 2005;87(1):37–45.

5. Sinha R, Rubash H. Extensor mechanism rupture. The adult knee. 1st ed. Philadelphia: Lippincott Williams & Wilkins; 2003. pp. 1351–8.
6. Ortiguera CJ, Berry DJ. Patellar fracture after total knee arthroplasty. J Bone Joint Surg. 2002;84(4):532–40.
7. Rand JA, Morrey BF, Bryan RS. Patellar tendon rupture after total knee arthroplasty. Clin Orthop Relat Res. 1989;244:233–8.
8. Emerson Jr RH, Head WC, Malinin TI. Reconstruction of patellar tendon rupture after total knee arthroplasty with an extensor mechanism allograft. Clin Orthop Relat Res. 1990;260:154–61.
9. Browne JA, Hanssen AD. Reconstruction of patellar tendon disruption after total knee arthroplasty: results of a new technique utilizing synthetic mesh. J Bone Joint Surg Am. 2011; 93(12):1137–43.
10. Leopold SS, Greidanus N, Paprosky WG, Berger RA, Rosenberg AG. High rate of failure of allograft reconstruction of the extensor mechanism after total knee arthroplasty. J Bone Joint Surg Am. 1999;81(11):1574–9.
11. Nazarian DG, Booth Jr RE. Extensor mechanism allografts in total knee arthroplasty. Clin Orthop Relat Res. 1999;367:123–9.
12. Burnett RS, Berger RA, Paprosky WG, Della Valle CJ, Jacobs JJ, Rosenberg AG. Extensor mechanism allograft reconstruction after total knee arthroplasty. A comparison of two techniques. J Bone Joint Surg Am. 2004;86-A(12):2694–9.

Recommended Reading

Springer BD. Acute and chronic patellar tendon ruptures after total knee arthroplasty. In: Techniques in revision hip and knee arthroplasty. 1st ed. St. Louis, MO: Elsevier Saunders; 2014. p. 204–11.

Springer BD, Della Valle CJ. Extensor mechanism allograft reconstruction after total knee arthroplasty. J Arthroplasty. 2008;23 (7 Suppl):35–8.

Chapter 11
Revision Total Knee Arthroplasty: Management of Periprosthetic Femur Fracture Around Total Knee Arthroplasty

Robert G.W. Girling V and Matthew C. Morrey

11.1 Introduction

Distal femur periprosthetic fractures are increasing in incidence and provide unique challenges for the orthopedic surgeon when considering treatment. The rates are reported between 0.3 % and 5.5 % in primary total knee replacements and up to 30 % in revised total knee replacements [1]. A majority of these fractures are low velocity mechanism in a patient with osteoporosis. The Rorabeck and Lewis classification not only provides a descriptive classification but also correlates with treatment options. These fractures are typically treated operatively due to importance of early mobilization on morbidity and mortality in this patient population. Type 1 and 2, implant stable fractures, can be fixed utilizing locked plating or intramedullary nailing while type 3, implant

R.G.W. GirlingV, MD (✉) • M.C. Morrey, MD
Department of Orthopedic Surgery, University of Texas
Health Science Center at San Antonio, 7703 Floyd Curl Drive,
San Antonio, TX 78229, USA
e-mail: Girling@uthscsa.edu

© Springer International Publishing Switzerland 2015   129
B.D. Springer and B.M. Curtin (eds.), *Complex Primary
and Revision Total Knee Arthroplasty: A Clinical Casebook*,
DOI 10.1007/978-3-319-18350-3_11

unstable, typically requires revision of femoral component. Operative fixation technique is based on soft tissue consider-ations, bone stock of distal fracture fragment, implant avail-ability, and other ipsilateral hardware or pathology present. Complexity of revision arthroplasty will depend on degree of comminution, previous implant type, ligamentous stability, and patient's functional level. As with any revision knee arthroplasty, technique should minimize bone removed and level of constraint should be appropriate for balance. Allograft combined with prosthesis or as an adjunct with internal fixa-tion is a consideration that can be useful when inadequate bone stock or healing potential is a concern. When treated appropriately, surgical intervention can facilitate early mobi-lization while leading to a high level of satisfaction.

11.1.1   Epidemiology

A majority of periprosthetic distal femur fractures are supra-condylar fractures. They happen more commonly due to low velocity falls in elderly patients rather than high velocity mechanisms which coincides with the biology and risk charac-teristics of the patient population. Risk factors described include revision arthroplasty, osteoporosis, rheumatoid arthri-tis, and chronic steroid use as with many fractures in older patients. Another often discussed risk factor for fracture is notching of the femur during the anterior cut of the distal femur. While biomechanics studies have confirmed that notch-ing weakens the interface above the femoral implant 18 % in bending and 39 % in torsion [2], other studies have not been able to correlate an increased clinical risk of fracture with notching [3]. It is generally agreed that notching should be avoided but is likely not the cause of most of these fractures.

11.1.2   Classification

Several classifications for distal femur periprosthetic frac-tures have been proposed. The one most commonly utilized is the Rorabeck and Taylor classification which takes into

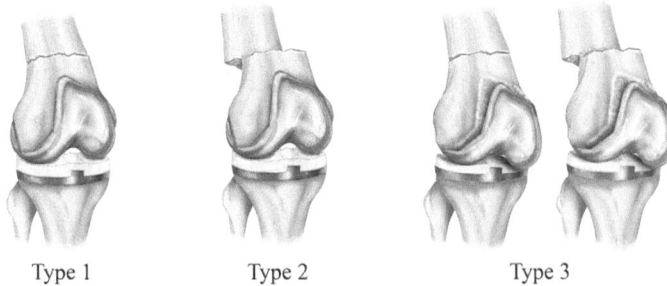

Type 1   Type 2   Type 3

Fig. 11.1. Rorabeck and Lewis classification: type 1 non-displaced fracture with well-fixed implant; type 2 displaced fracture with well-fixed implant; type 3 non-displaced or displaced fracture with loose implant.

account both fracture location and implant stability [4] (see Fig. 11.1).

Type 1: Non-displaced and well-fixed implant
Type 2: Displaced and well-fixed implant
Type 3: Non-displaced or displaced with loose implant

11.1.3 Management

Treatment options for distal femur periprosthetic fractures include nonoperative treatment, conventional plate fixation, locking plate fixation, intramedullary nail, external fixation, and revision knee arthroplasty. Nonoperative treatment is typically not advised unless surgery is medically contraindicated. Nonoperative management often leads to high rates of nonunion, malunion, and poor patient satisfaction [5, 6]. External fixation may be a reasonable option in some patients but requires pins to be placed away from the total knee implants given high incidence of pin site infection. This typically requires spanning the knee joint which does not facilitate early motion and contributes to a stiff knee. For these reasons open reduction and internal fixation versus revision arthroplasty are the treatments of choice in distal femur periprosthetic fractures.

The following cases below will discuss the indications for plate fixation, intramedullary nailing, and revision knee arthroplasty.

11.2   Case Presentation #1

A 66-year-old woman presented to the emergency department with right thigh pain and deformity after slipping on a rock while cleaning her pond. She had previous total knee replacement 7 years prior with previously well-functioning and pain-free result. She denies any other injuries. Her comorbidities include morbid obesity, type 2 diabetes, chronic kidney disease, hypertension, and hyperlipidemia.

Physical exam shows isolated pain and deformity to the distal femur with skin intact. Previous surgical wound is well healed with no evidence of skin compromise and leg is neurovascularly intact. Patient is morbidly obese with much of her weight carried in her thigh.

11.2.1   Diagnosis/Assessment

The patient has a closed distal femur periprosthetic fracture with a stable implant, Lewis and Rorabeck type 2 fracture. The displaced component is meta-diaphyseal with a non-displaced fracture extension ending at the level of the implant (see Fig. 11.2).

11.2.2   Management

The recommended treatment options for this patient include locking distal femur plate vs. a retrograde intramedullary implant. Both have been shown to provide superior fixation when compared to traditional nonlocking plates [7, 8]. In this case we chose to use an intramedullary nail. The intramedullary nail requires a smaller exposure which is a concern in this obese patient with multiple comorbidities. It also allows

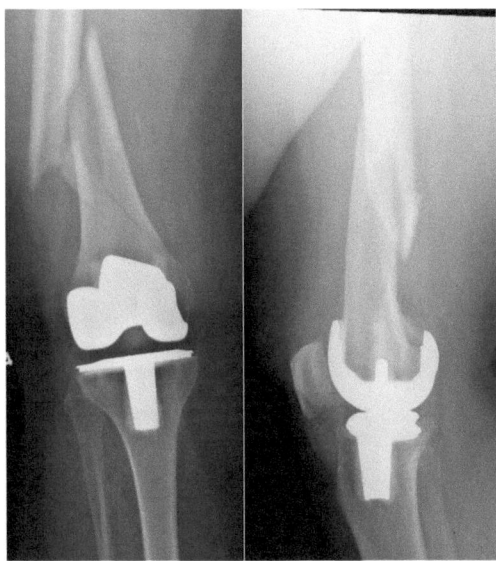

Fig. 11.2. Displaced distal femur periprosthetic fracture with likely stable implant, type 2, with a non-displaced fracture extension ending at level of implant.

distribution of forces over a longer construct in a fracture that extends into the diaphyseal region of the femur [8]. Some studies have shown lower nonunion rates in intramedullary nails when compared to locking plates [9, 10]. Considerations that should be made for an intramedullary nail include adequate bone stock distal to fracture for locking screws, a stable implant, and an implant that will facilitate nail insertion. Relative contraindications include hip hardware (i.e., existing intramedullary nail proximally) or existing hip arthritis that may require hip arthroplasty in the near future. In these cases, retrograde intramedullary implant may be possible if there is an adequate amount of space between the distal tip of any existing fixation in the proximal femur and the proximal tip of retrograde fixation so as not to create a stress riser.

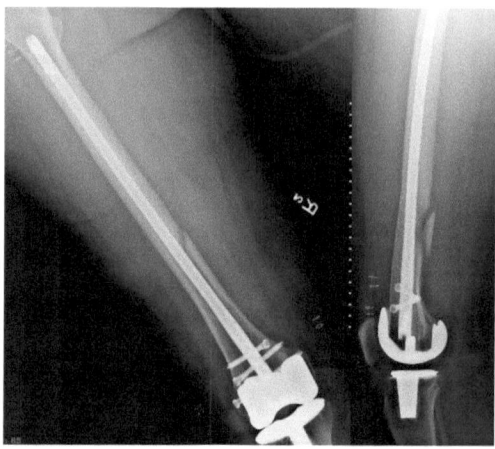

FIG. 11.3. Type 2 distal femur periprosthetic fracture after reduction and internal fixation with a retrograde intramedullary nail.

A retrograde intramedullary nail was placed through the intercondylar notch through small portion of previous skin exposure. Careful consideration was taken to protect the polyethylene and femoral component with the soft tissue protector. The nail was then placed in a standard manner. Appropriately sized nail was inserted and locked with 2 screws proximally and 3 screws distally. Patient was made weight bearing as tolerated in the immediately postoperative period (see Fig. 11.3).

11.2.3 Clinical Pearls/Pitfalls

- Rorabeck type 1 or 2 fractures
- No previous hip arthroplasty or hip arthritis
- Adequate bone stock distal to fracture site
- Distal femur implant facilitates intramedullary nail
- Skin over knee facilitates insertion
- Femoral radius of curvature appropriate for insertion point accessibility, heavily influenced by both fixation nail and current arthroplasty implant.

11.3   Case Presentation #2

The patient is a 63-year-old female presented to the emergency department after trip and fall with left thigh pain and deformity. She had previous total knee replacement 6 months ago and was doing well walking without a walking aid prior to the fall. Patient denies any other injuries. Medical problems include hypertension, diabetes, and asthma.

Physical exam shows isolated pain and deformity to the distal femur with skin intact. Previous surgical wound is well healed with no evidence of skin compromise and leg is neurovascularly intact.

11.3.1   Diagnosis/Assessment

The patient has a closed distal femur periprosthetic fracture with a stable implant, Lewis and Rorabeck type 2 fracture. Fracture is at the level of the anterior femoral interface with mild comminution and transverse (see Fig. 11.4).

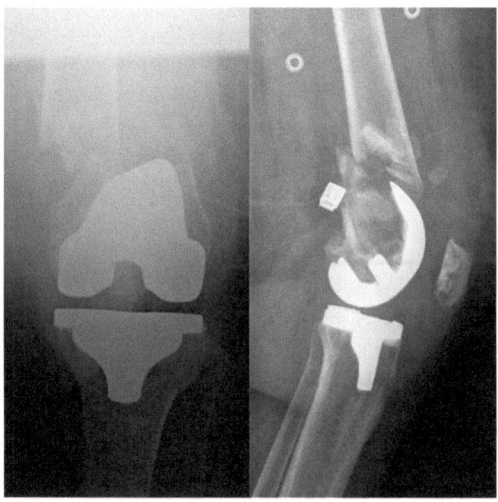

Fig. 11.4. Displaced distal femur periprosthetic fracture with likely stable implant, type 2, transverse with mild comminution.

11.3.2   Management

The recommended treatment options for this patient include locking distal femur plate, retrograde intramedullary implant, or revision knee arthroplasty. Intraoperative assessment of the distal femur component is necessary to ensure that it remains well fixed. If it does remain well fixed, it appears that adequate bone stock to avoid a revision knee replacement. An intramedullary implant is not a great option due to distal fracture location which will not accommodate adequate distal locking screws. A locking distal femur plate has been shown to be an effective treatment option for this fracture and is superior to nonlocking plates which have significantly higher rates of malunion, nonunion, and reoperation rates [7]. Allograft may be utilized as an adjunct to distal femur plating [11] or even intramedullary fixation [12], when additional stability or biology may be required. The use of allograft strut fixation either alone, or in conjunction with plate and/or intramedullary fixation, is largely surgeon preference but has been shown to provide reliable fracture union, improved alignment, and increased femoral bone stock with a high incorporation rate [13].

A distal femur locking plate was chosen for fixation of the fracture. A lateral approach was made to the distal femur, and the distal femur implant to bone interface was visualized to confirm the component remained well fixed. After confirming implant stability, the fracture was reduced and the plate was placed using AO technique. Proximal screws were placed percutaneously with the aid of fluoroscopy to minimize soft tissue disruption. No allograft was utilized based on clinical judgement in this patient. The patient was non-weight bearing for 2 weeks and progressive weight bearing for next 4 weeks (see Fig. 11.5).

11.3.3   Clinical Pearls/Pitfalls

- Rorabeck type 1 or 2 fractures
- Adequate bone stock distal to fracture site
- Consider allograft extracortical or intramedullary
- Locking plates are preferable to nonlocking plates

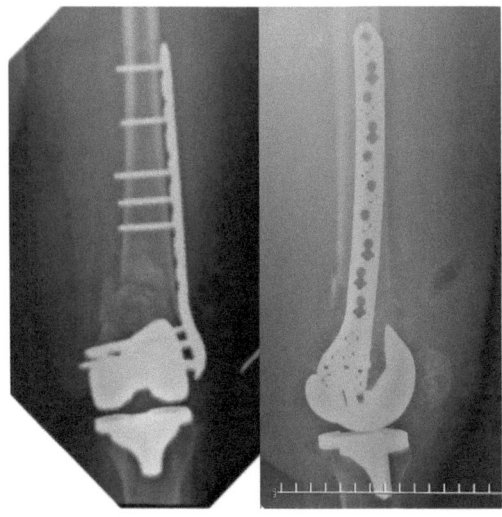

F<small>IG</small>. 11.5. Type 2 distal femur periprosthetic fracture after open reduction and internal fixation with distal femur plate.

11.4   Case Presentation #3

The patient is a 76-year-old female presenting to the emergency department after slipping in water and falling from standing. She now presents with severe knee pain and deformity. She previously underwent total knee arthroplasty 2 years prior to injury with good pain relief and function. Patient denies any other injuries and medical comorbidities include hypertension, hyperlipidemia, and cardiac disease with previous intervention.

11.4.1   Diagnosis/Assessment

The patient has a closed displaced distal femur periprosthetic fracture but unclear whether implant is stable, Lewis and Rorabeck type 2 vs. 3 (see Fig. 11.6). A CT scan was obtained

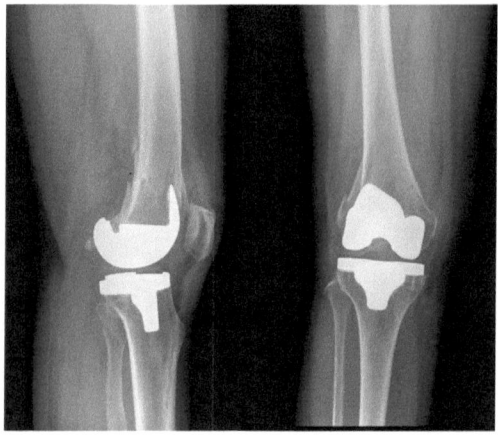

FIG. 11.6. Displaced distal femur periprosthetic fracture with suspected loose implant, type 2 vs. 3.

which shows the comminution extends to the implant bone interface indicating the implant will likely be unstable but unable to tell for certain with imaging alone (see Fig. 11.7).

11.4.2   Management

The recommended treatment options will depend on whether the implant is found to be stable intraoperatively. If the implant is stable, a distal femur locking plate may be a good option. In this case however, it is likely that the implant is unstable and will require revision arthroplasty. The type of prosthesis used is determined based on bone stock and patient activity level (i.e., minimal ambulators, who may rely on their implants largely for transfers only, versus more active, mobile patients who may be household or community ambulators). When adequate metaphyseal bone stock is present, revision techniques related to deficient bone stock may be utilized including stemmed implants and augments. Often inadequate metaphyseal bone stock is present and either

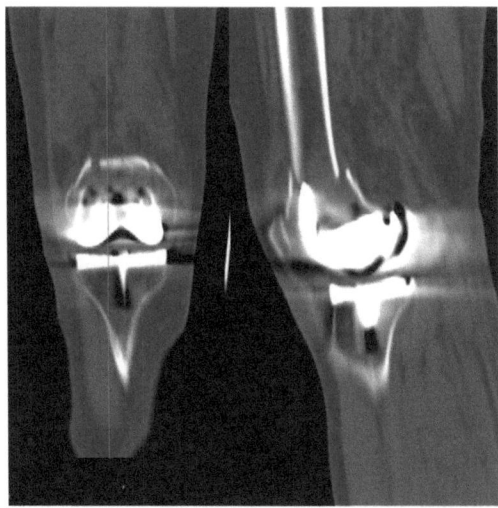

Fig. 11.7. CT scan of the displaced distal femur periprosthetic fracture seen in Fig. 11.6 that confirms comminution extends to implant bone interface and will likely be loose, type 3, which assists with preoperative planning.

structural allograft or a distal femur replacement is required. Combined distal femur allograft with stemmed implant has been reported with ability to reattach host tissues with good results [14]. Distal femur replacement with hinged prosthesis also provides a reliable option but is best suited in low demand patients [15, 16].

The fracture was assessed intraoperatively and determined that the implant was not well fixed. Fracture comminution extended into the metaphysis making revision arthroplasty with augments or stemmed implants inadequate. Based on the patient's low functional demands and comorbidities, a distal femur replacement with hinged prosthesis was utilized. The patient was made weight bearing as tolerated and progressed well after surgery (see Fig. 11.8).

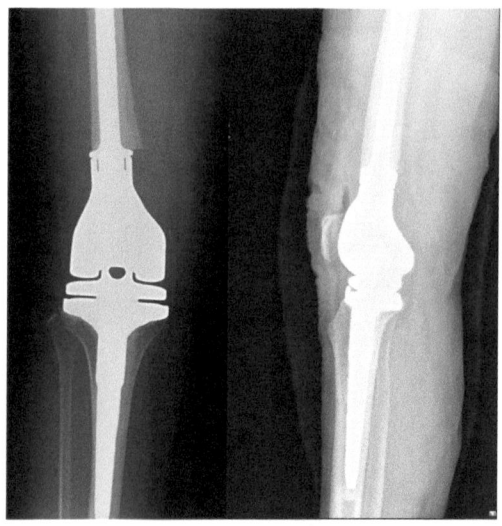

FIG. 11.8. Type 3 distal femur periprosthetic fracture after revision arthroplasty with a distal femur replacement due to severity and level of fracture comminution.

11.4.3   Clinical Pearls/Pitfalls

- Rorabeck type 3 fractures
- Implant choice based on bone stock and activity level
- Revision principles apply; i.e., appropriate implants available, struts and/or plates available, assessment of bone stock intraoperatively, and appropriate exposure planned.
- Favor less constraint and preserve bone in young/active
- Favor one surgery, short operative time, early mobility in old/inactive

References

1. Della Rocca GJ, Leung KS, Pape H-C. Periprosthetic fractures: epidemiology and future projections. J Orthop Trauma. 2011;25 Suppl 2(6):S66–70.
2. Lesh ML, Schneider DJ, Deol G, Davis B, Jacobs CR, Pellegrini VD. The consequences of anterior femoral notching in total knee

arthroplasty. A biomechanical study. J Bone Joint Surg Am. 2000;82-A(8):1096–101.

3. Ritter MA, Thong AE, Keating EM, Faris PM, Meding JB, Berend ME, Pierson MD, Kenneth DE. The effect of femoral notching during total knee arthroplasty on the prevalence of postoperative femoral fractures and on clinical outcome. J Bone Joint Surg Am. 2005;87(11):2411–4.

4. Rorabeck CH, Taylor JW. Periprosthetic fractures of the femur complicating total knee arthroplasty. Orthop Clin North Am. 1999;30(2):265–77.

5. Culp RW. Supracondylar fracture of the femur following prosthetic knee arthroplasty. Clin Orthop Relat Res. 1987;222: 212–22.

6. Su ET, DeWal H, Di Cesare PE. Periprosthetic femoral fractures above total knee replacements. J Am Acad Orthop Surg. 2004; 12(1):12–20.

7. Herrera DA, Kregor PJ, Cole PA, Levy BA, Jönsson A, Zlowodzki M. Treatment of acute distal femur fractures above a total knee arthroplasty: systematic review of 415 cases (1981-2006). Acta Orthop. 2008;79(1):22–7.

8. Bong MR, Egol K, Koval KJ, Kummer FJ, Su ET, Iesaka K, Bayer J, Di Cesare PE. Comparison of the LISS and a retrograde-inserted supracondylar intramedullary nail for fixation of a periprosthetic distal femur fracture proximal to a total knee arthroplasty. J Arthroplasty. 2002;17(7):876–81.

9. Meneghini RM, Keyes BJ, Reddy KK, Maar DC. Modern retrograde intramedullary nails versus periarticular locked plates for supracondylar femur fractures after total knee arthroplasty. J Arthroplasty. 2014;29(7):1478–81.

10. Large TM, Kellam JF, Bosse MJ, Sims SH, Althausen P, Masonis JL. Locked plating of supracondylar periprosthetic femur fractures. J Arthroplasty. 2008;23(6 Suppl 1):115–20.

11. Wang JW, Wang CJ. Supracondylar fractures of the femur above total knee arthroplasties with cortical allograft struts. J Arthroplasty. 2002;17:365–72.

12. Tani Y, Inoue K, Kaneko H, Nishioka J, Hukuda S. Intramedullary fibular graft for supracondylar fracture of the femur following total knee arthroplasty. Arch Orthop Trauma Surg. 1998; 117:103–4.

13. Haddad FS, Duncan CP, Berry DJ, Lewallen DG, Gross AE, Chandler HP. Periprosthetic femoral fractures around well-fixed implants: use of cortical onlay allografts with or without a plate. J Bone Joint Surg Am. 2002;84-A(6):945–50.

14. Kraay MJ, Goldberg VM, Figgie MP, Figgie 3rd HE. Distal femoral replacement with allograft/prosthetic reconstruction for treatment of supracondylar fractures in patients with total knee arthroplasty. J Arthroplasty. 1992;7:7–16.
15. Jassim SS, McNamara I, Hopgood P. Distal femoral replacement in periprosthetic fracture around total knee arthroplasty. Injury. 2014;45(3):550–3.
16. Saidi K, Ben-Lulu O, Tsuji M, Safir O, Gross AE, Backstein D. Supracondylar periprosthetic fractures of the knee in the elderly patients: a comparison of treatment using allograft-implant composites, standard revision components, distal femoral replacement prosthesis. J Arthroplasty. 2014;29(1):110–4.

Chapter 12
Revision Total Knee Arthroplasty: Management of Bone Loss

Robert M. Molloy and Nicholas T. Ting

12.1 Case Presentation

A 69-year-old man, otherwise active and healthy, presented to clinic with a 1-year history of a painful right total knee arthroplasty (TKA), worse in the last 6 months. Pain was worse with activity, although he was able to ambulate for ten blocks without the use of any assist devices. He denied any precipitating trauma or injury, as well as any constitutional symptoms or history of painful TKA. Past history revealed staged, bilateral total knee arthroplasties performed approximately 15–20 years prior. He stated that up until 1 year ago, he had had an otherwise unremarkable postoperative course. Physical examination of his right knee revealed no effusion, warmth, or erythema; his previous midline incision was well healed. He demonstrated some pain with active range of motion from 5° to 130°, as well as increased varus/valgus laxity. Routine radiographs revealed bilateral TKAs with signs of significant osteolysis, component loosening, and subsidence (Fig. 12.1). Right knee X-rays demonstrated a cruciate retaining cemented, modular TKA with loosening of the

R.M. Molloy, MD (✉) • N.T. Ting, MD
Department of Orthopedic Surgery, Cleveland Clinic,
9500 Euclid Avenue, Cleveland, OH 44195, USA
e-mail: molloyr@ccf.org

© Springer International Publishing Switzerland 2015   143
B.D. Springer and B.M. Curtin (eds.), *Complex Primary and Revision Total Knee Arthroplasty: A Clinical Casebook*,
DOI 10.1007/978-3-319-18350-3_12

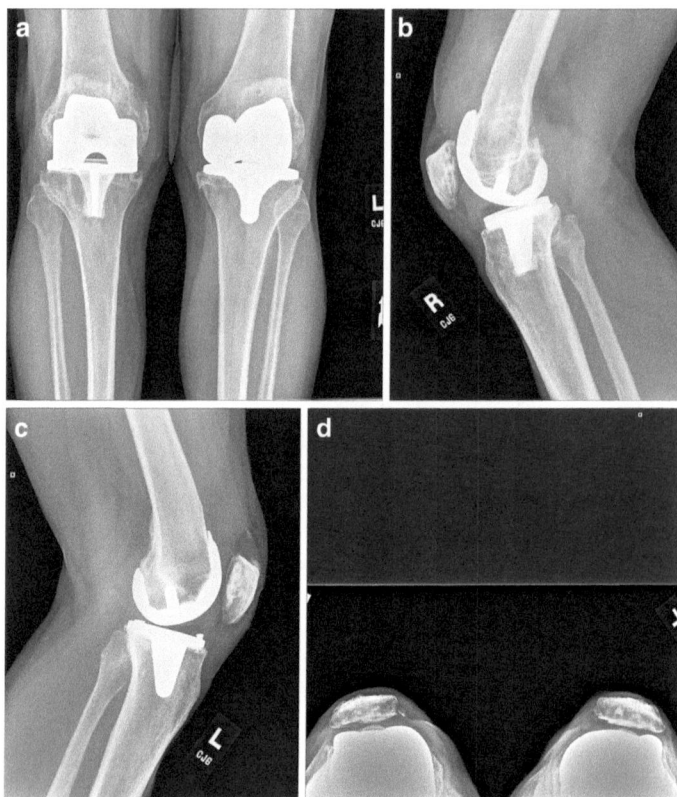

FIG. 12.1. (**a–d**) Preoperative X-rays reveal a cemented right and left total knee arthroplasties with radiographic signs of loosening. The right TKA tibial component has subsided into varus.

femoral and tibial components, the latter having subsided into varus; there were significant osteolytic lesions surrounding both components. While there was no distinct metal-line sign present [1], there was radiographic densification of the periarticular soft tissue seen on the lateral view. Of note, left knee X-rays revealed a similar pattern. Serum erythrocyte sedimentation rate (ESR) and C-reactive protein (CRP) were 1 mm/h (normal range, 0–15 mm/h) and 0.1 mg/dL (normal range, 0.0–1.0 mg/dL), respectively. Serum cobalt and chromium levels were elevated to 12 μg/L (normal range, <1.0) and 3.9 μg/L (normal range, 0.2–0.6).

12.1.1 Diagnosis/Assessment

The patient presented with a chronically painful right TKA and late instability in the setting of elevated serum metal ion levels, and hence was presumed to have full-thickness polyethylene wear and resultant osteolysis. The index of suspicion for this was high on the left knee as well, but our work-up and treatment focused on his symptomatic right TKA. Chronic, indolent periprosthetic infection could not be ruled out either, but his history, physical exam, and laboratory results suggested an aseptic etiology; hence, a preoperative knee aspiration for synovial analysis was deferred in lieu of an intraoperative assessment. Historically, polyethylene wear and its sequelae (aseptic loosening, osteolysis, late instability) are common causes for revision total knee arthroplasty, particularly with the use of modular tibial components. In fact, osteolysis induced by wear debris of ultra-high-molecular-weight polyethylene emerged as a significant problem, presumably related to backside polyethylene wear as well as poor quality polyethylene (i.e., gamma irradiated in air). While a rare cause of failure after total knee arthroplasty, metallosis was also considered in this case given the significant osteolysis, joint space narrowing, and radiographic densification of the periarticular soft tissue seen radiographically [2]. Metallosis has only previously been reported when there has been abnormal metal-on-metal contact, and we suspected this phenomenon here, prompting our preoperative interest in serum metal ion levels.

12.1.2 Management

In a patient with presumed metallosis, osteolysis, and aseptic loosening due to full-thickness polyethylene wear, revision TKA involving all components must be discussed. In particular, the

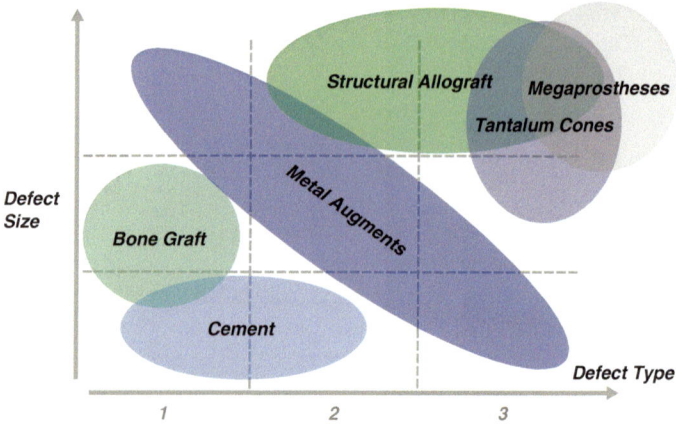

Fig. 12.2. Matrix of bone loss filling options in revision TKA. *X*-axis represents the relative defect size, while the *y*-axis represents the defect type, according to the Anderson Orthopedic Research Institute (AORI) classification.

method of reconstruction depends on the remaining bone stock, ligamentous integrity, and the ability to balance flexion/extension gaps. The Anderson Orthopedic Research Institute (AORI) classification grades bone loss associated with revision TKA based on defect size and the degree of metaphyseal involvement [3]. This provides a useful guide for predicting the options for reconstruction. Cement, morselized allograft, or metal augments can be individually used to fill smaller, confined defects (<1 cm). As the defect size or degree of metaphyseal involvement increases, reconstruction may require impaction grafting, structural allograft, metaphyseal sleeves, porous metal cones, composite allograft, megaprostheses, or some combination of any of these modalities (Fig. 12.2). While preoperative radiographs can predict the anticipated bone loss, they often underestimate the actual bone loss encountered intraoperatively [4]. Hence, adequate preoperative planning means anticipating the use of any combination of the aforementioned defect-filling modalities.

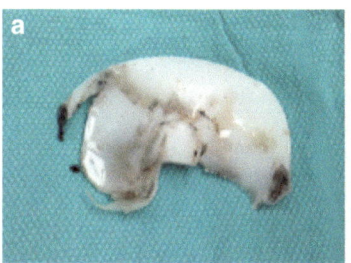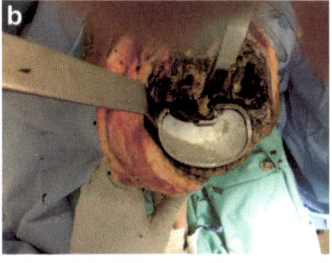

Fɪɢ. 12.3. There is full-thickness wear of the polyethylene insert, most prominently on the posterolateral corner (**a**), and a corresponding completely worn corner of the tibial base plate beneath it (**b**).

12.1.3 Outcome

The patient underwent elective revision TKA after thorough discussion about the potential bone loss and the spectrum of possible treatment options; while less likely, the potentials for underlying periprosthetic infection and two-stage revision were also discussed. At the time of surgery, there was extensive metallosis and metallic debris, but intraoperative frozen sections were unremarkable for acute inflammation. On gross examination, the all-polyethylene patellar button was frankly loose, and there was significant femoral component burnishing. There was full-thickness wear of the polyethylene insert, most prominently on the posterolateral corner, and a corresponding completely worn corner of the tibial base plate beneath it (Fig. 12.3). Removal of all hardware revealed significant osteolysis of both the distal femur and proximal tibia with type III bone defects, as classified by the AORI scale. On the femoral side, only a shell of bone remained medially, with a significant osteolytic defect on the lateral side as well (Fig. 12.4a). On the tibial side, there was a significant osteolytic defect centrally (Fig. 12.4b). The femoral defect was filled with a trabecular metal distal femoral cone and a press-fit stem, along with bilateral distal femoral and posterior augments (Fig. 12.5a). Likewise, the tibial defect was addressed with a trabecular metal cone with a press-fit

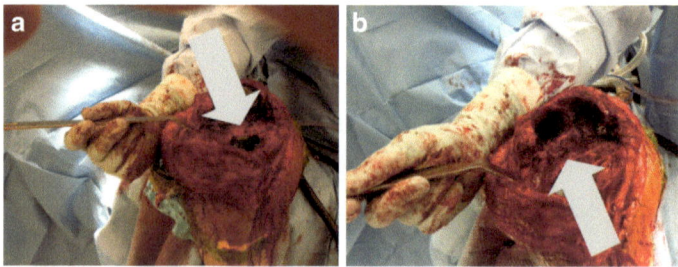

Fig. 12.4. In the femur, there is only a shell of bone remaining on the medial side and a significant osteolytic defect laterally (**a**). There is a significant osteolytic defect centrally seen in the tibia (**b**).

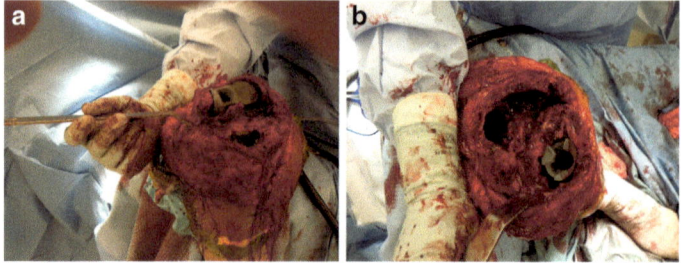

Fig. 12.5. Trabecular metal cones are seen filling defects in the distal femur (**a**) and proximal tibia (**b**).

stem and bilateral tibial augments (Fig. 12.5b). A total stabilized insert was used to address ligamentous instability. Postoperatively, the patient was restricted to 20 lbs-weight bearing for 6 weeks in a hinged knee brace, locked from 0° to 90°. At his 8-week postoperative follow-up visit, he was already weight bearing as tolerated without a brace and demonstrated an active range of motion from 0° to 130°. He did complain of some new-onset, mid-shaft tibial pain, which was mild in nature and unrelated to any injury or other symptoms. His radiographs demonstrated stemmed femoral and tibial components in good overall alignment (Fig. 12.6). There was no evidence of fracture or loosening, and we attributed this pain to modulus mismatch with the press-fit tibial stem.

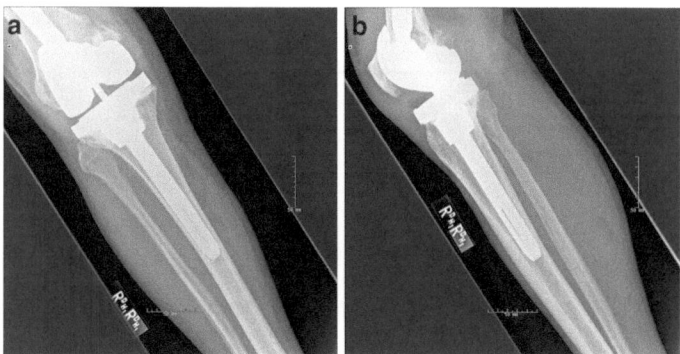

FIG. 12.6. Postoperative week 8 AP (**a**) and lateral (**b**) radiographs demonstrate stemmed femoral and tibial components in good overall alignment.

12.2 Literature Review

Bone loss is a common problem in revision total knee arthroplasty. In this case, the extensive bone loss was a result of osteolysis secondary to polyethylene wear and metallosis; however, the etiology of bone deficiency can also include aseptic loosening resulting in direct mechanical bone loss, septic loosening, instability stress shielding, or iatrogenic during implant removal. No two revisions are the same. As the type of bone loss can be highly variable in each case, so too are the potential reconstruction options.

In the management of bone loss, it is important to consider defect size and location, as well as patient-specific characteristics such as age, life expectancy, body mass index, and activity level. As aforementioned, one widely used method for categorizing defects based on size and metaphyseal involvement is the AORI classification outlined by Engh. Type 1 defects involve an intact metaphyseal rim and joint line with bone defects of less than 1 cm; these defects can be reconstituted with cement, morselized allograft, or metal augments. Type 2 defects involve significant cancellous bone loss with a

TABLE 12.1. Management of bone loss in revision total knee arthroplasty.

Defect type	Defect size	Treatment options
Contained	<5 mm	PMMA fill
	5–10 mm	Reinforced PMMA
	>10 mm	Morselized allograft or porous metal augments
Non-contained	<5 mm	PMMA
	5–10 mm, <50 % femoral condyle/tibial plateau	Reinforced PMMA
	5–15 mm, >50 % femoral condyle/tibial plateau	TKA modular systems with stems, augments
	>15 mm	Structural allografts; megaprostheses, or porous metal augments

Abbreviations: *PMMA* polymethylmethacrylate (acrylic bone cement), *TKA* total knee arthroplasty

relatively intact metaphyseal rim and require joint line restoration; these defects are further categorized into type 2a (only one femoral condyle or one side of the tibial plateau involved) and type 2b (both femoral condyles or both sides of the tibial plateau involved). Reconstruction options for type 2 defects include metal augments, impaction grafting, structural allograft, metaphyseal sleeves, or porous metal cones. Type 3 defects involve large metaphyseal rim defects with extensive cancellous bone loss; reconstruction options include impaction grafting, structural allograft, metaphyseal sleeves, porous metal cones, composite allograft, or mega-prostheses. Another classification scheme, outlined by Clatworthy and Gross (Table 12.1), categorizes defects initially as contained or non-contained. Defects can be further stratified as type I—contained with metaphyseal bone intact, in which restoration of the joint line does not require bone grafting or augmentation; type II—contained with compromised metaphyseal bone and requiring bone grafting, cement fill, or augments to restore the joint line; type III—non-contained, noncircumferential defects requiring a femoral head allograft, partial distal femur, or partial proximal tibia; and type IV—non-contained, circumferential defects requiring a segmental distal femoral or proximal tibial graft.

The armamentarium of treatment options for bone loss is extensive, including polymethylmethacrylate (PMMA) with or without reinforcing screws, autograft, morselized or structural allograft [5], modular TKA systems including stems, wedges and metal augments, and orthopedic salvage systems such as mega- or tumor prostheses [6]. For reconstitution of contained defects, morselized allograft is better suited than structural allograft and may be associated with a higher rate of incorporation. However, the drawbacks of allograft use include late resorption, fracture or nonunion in the case of structural allograft, and risk of disease transmission. Other alternatives to small, contained defects include filling with PMMA, reinforced with one or more screws if the defect is larger enough. Metallic augments available with modular TKA systems can also be used to address areas of discrete bone loss.

12.2.1 Ultraporous Metals

Ultraporous metals fabricated into augments and cones, such as those used in this patient, are helpful innovations for addressing larger structural defects in revision TKA [7–9]. While there is a paucity of information in the literature regarding the long-term outcomes of these reconstruction options, short-term results have been promising. Meneghini et al. [10] reported on the use of porous tantalum augments for treatment of extensive tibial bone loss in a series of 15 revision TKAs (15 patients) that included seven AORI type 2B and eight type 3 defects. At a mean follow-up of 34 months, all cases went on to osseointegration without loosening or migration. More recently, Huang et al. prospectively followed 83 knees that underwent revision TKA with metaphyseal sleeves [11], including 36 sleeves used in femoral revisions and 83 sleeves in tibial revisions. At a mean follow-up of 2.4 years, none of the implants demonstrated progressive radiolucency around the metaphyseal sleeves, and only two (2.7 %) patients required revision for aseptic loosening of their tibial components.

12.2.2   Salvage Prostheses

As bone loss becomes more severe, both in size and containment, revision options expand to include tumor-type megaprostheses [6]. Distal femoral replacements have been utilized for a variety of indications, ranging from severely comminuted periprosthetic fractures compromising implant fixation to catastrophic revision scenarios involving severe osteolysis, septic failure, or ligamentous instability. Berend et al. reported on a series of 38 distal femoral replacements in 36 patients with a mean follow-up of 33 months [6]. The most common indications were periprosthetic fracture (32 %), septic failure (21 %), and aseptic loosening (18 %). The average size of bone loss encountered was 7 cm. Complications included two deaths within 3 months of surgery and three reoperations—two for recurrent infection and one for periprosthetic fracture.

In their review of the literature, Lombardi et al. offered an algorithmic approach to managing bone loss in revision TKA [12]. PMMA cement alone can be used for bone defects <5 mm in size. For deficits of 5–10 mm and <50 % of the femoral condyle or tibial plateau, PMMA with reinforcing screws is recommended. Morselized allograft can be used to fill contained deficits >5 mm. For non-contained defects 5–15 mm and >50 % of the femoral condyle and tibial plateau, they recommend modular TKA systems with stems and augments. And in the case of non-contained deficits >15 mm, structural allografts, tumor-type megaprostheses, and porous metal augments provide suitable options.

12.3 Clinical Pearls/Pitfalls

- Bone loss is a common problem in revision total knee arthroplasty.
- Metallosis must be considered in the setting of the chronically painful TKA with radiographic signs of osteolysis and component loosening.
- While preoperative radiographs can predict the anticipated bone loss, they often underestimate the actual bone loss encountered intraoperatively.
- Preoperative and intraoperative classification of bone deficiency can predict the options for reconstruction.
- As there is a spectrum of bone-filling options, reconstitution of bone defects often involves more than one modality of treatment.
- At short-term follow-up, revision TKA with each of the different modes of bone reconstitution provides reliable fixation.

References

1. Weissman BN, Scott RD, Brick GW, Corson JM. Radiographic detection of metal-induced synovitis as a complication of arthroplasty of the knee. J Bone Joint Surg Am. 1991;73:1002–7.
2. Romesburg JW, Wasserman PL, Schoppe CH. Metallosis and metal-induced synovitis following total knee arthroplasty: review of radiographic and CT findings. J Radiol Case Rep. 2010;4: 7–17.
3. Engh GA, Ammeen DJ. Bone loss with revision total knee arthroplasty: defect classification and alternatives for reconstruction. Instr Course Lect. 1999;48:167–75.
4. Mulhall KJ, Ghomrawi HM, Engh GA, Clark CR, Lotke P, Saleh KJ. Radiographic prediction of intraoperative bone loss in knee arthroplasty revision. Clin Orthop Relat Res. 2006;446:51–8.
5. Burnett RS, Keeney JA, Maloney WJ, Clohisy JC. Revision total knee arthroplasty for major osteolysis. Iowa Orthop J. 2009;29: 28–37.
6. Berend KR, Lombardi Jr AV. Distal femoral replacement in nontumor cases with severe bone loss and instability. Clin Orthop Relat Res. 2009;467:485–92.

7. Radnay CS, Scuderi GR. Management of bone loss: augments, cones, offset stems. Clin Orthop Relat Res. 2006;446:83–92.
8. Patil N, Lee K, Goodman SB. Porous tantalum in hip and knee reconstructive surgery. J Biomed Mater Res B Appl Biomater. 2009;89:242–51.
9. Levine B, Sporer S, Della Valle CJ, Jacobs JJ, Paprosky W. Porous tantalum in reconstructive surgery of the knee: a review. J Knee Surg. 2007;20:185–94.
10. Meneghini RM, Lewallen DG, Hanssen AD. Use of porous tantalum metaphyseal cones for severe tibial bone loss during revision total knee replacement. Surgical technique. J Bone Joint Surg Am. 2009;91 Suppl 2 Pt 1:131–8.
11. Huang R, Barrazueta G, Ong A, et al. Revision total knee arthroplasty using metaphyseal sleeves at short-term follow-up. Orthopedics. 2014;37:e804–9.
12. Lombardi AV, Berend KR, Adams JB. Management of bone loss in revision TKA: it's a changing world. Orthopedics. 2010;33:662.

Chapter 13
Revision Total Knee Arthroplasty: Management of Ligamentous Instability

Colin A. Mudrick and Brian M. Curtin

13.1 Introduction

Instability after total knee arthroplasty is second only to infection as a cause for revision within the first 5 years [1]. As the numbers of knee arthroplasties performed in the United States grow at a steady rate, this clinical problem will likely increase accordingly. In managing these patients, it is critical to identify a clear etiology before proceeding with revision surgery. Preoperative planning is also essential to ensure that all necessary implants are available. While the best solution to this problem is prevention, these cases do provide insight into potentially avoidable mistakes at the time of primary surgery. There are however unavoidable circumstances that can lead to this problem, and it is important to be familiar with current techniques and available equipment necessary to manage such cases.

C.A. Mudrick, MD • B.M. Curtin, MD, MS (✉)
OrthoCarolina Hip and Knee Center, Charlotte, NC, USA
e-mail: brian.curtin@orthocarolina.com

© Springer International Publishing Switzerland 2015   155
B.D. Springer and B.M. Curtin (eds.), *Complex Primary and Revision Total Knee Arthroplasty: A Clinical Casebook*, DOI 10.1007/978-3-319-18350-3_13

13.2   Case Presentation

A 62-year-old male with history of a right total knee arthroplasty 2 years prior presented to the office with continued pain with range of motion and activity. He described a sensation of giving way or collapse of the knee at times, particularly with stair descent. The patient also complained of occasional increased warmth in the knee and associated recurrent effusions. He denied fevers or chills and did not recall any problems with wound healing following his surgery. He felt that he had lost some of his motion in the right knee over the past year. On physical examination the patient ambulated with a mild right-sided antalgic gait with no assist device. Examination of the right knee revealed a mild effusion with slight warmth to palpation. Tenderness was elicited over the lateral joint line and in the area of the pes bursae at the proximal medial tibia. Range of motion was from 0 to 105° with pain at the extremes of motion. The knee was stable to valgus stress but had mild laxity with varus stress in full extension and 30° of flexion. There was at least 5 mm of opening to varus stress on the lateral side of the knee in 90° of flexion and increased AP translation with the patient seated and knee hanging at 90° of flexion with AP stress.

Although ESR and CRP were normal at 8 and 0.2 respectively, concerns clinically for potential infection led to aspiration of the knee. Knee aspirate in the office resulted in 30 mL of bloody synovial fluid and WBC count of 450 with high red blood cell count.

Cultures were no growth at 14 days.

Radiographs taken in the office and review of the previous operative report confirmed a cemented posterior stabilized total knee arthroplasty with a rotating platform polyethylene insert and resurfaced patella. A slight radiolucency behind the anterior flange of the femur was noted but otherwise components appeared well fixed. A slightly asymmetrical patellar cut was observed with lateral tilt on the Merchant view (Fig. 13.1).

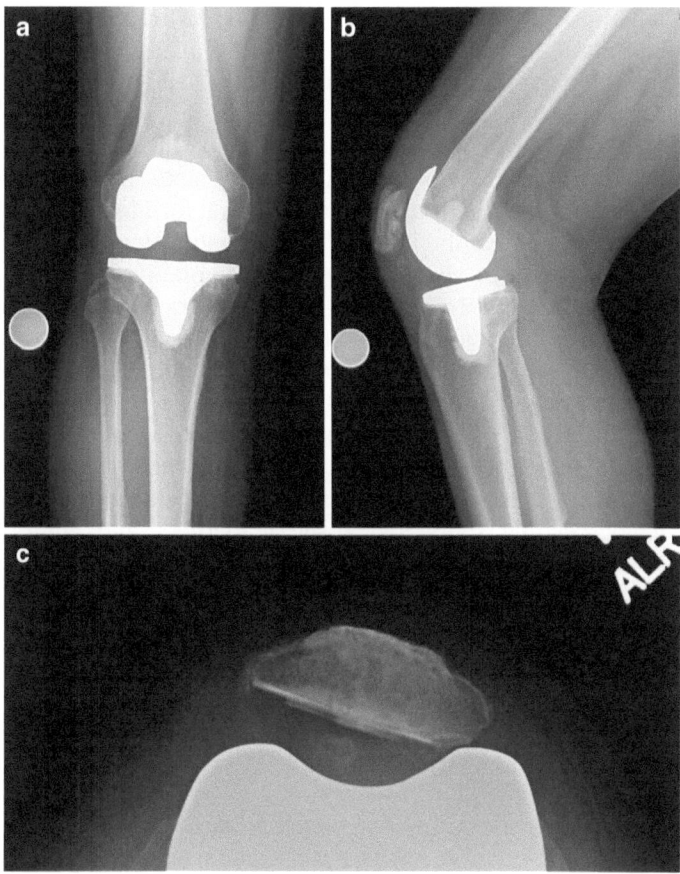

FIG. 13.1. Preoperative AP (**a**), lateral (**b**), and Merchant view (**c**) radiographs demonstrating component positioning after index TKA procedure.

13.3 Diagnosis/Assessment

13.3.1 History

The evaluation of ligamentous instability after total knee arthroplasty continues to be challenging, particularly in cases when radiographic and/or physical exam findings are not inherently obvious. As always, a detailed history both before and after the index procedure is vital. Patients with subtle instability patterns complain of catching, giving way, or anterior knee pain. Anterior knee pain often occurs as the patient tries to stabilize their knee by firing the quadriceps muscle on a chronic basis. While not always available, preoperative radiographs, exam findings, and indication for the initial procedure can be helpful in these circumstances. Important considerations also include type of implant, a detailed postoperative course including physical therapy reports, pain chronology, operative technique including ligamentous releases, and pertinent patient factors including history of neuromuscular or connective tissue disease [2, 3]. Additional risk factors that have been described include obesity as well as planovalgus foot deformities [3]. Other historical clues in subtle cases include recurrent effusion, difficulty with ascending/descending stairs, soft tissue tenderness, and anterior knee pain [4]. Implant migration and failure, neuromotor dysfunction, and extensor mechanism failure are other potential rare causes of global instability. Symptoms include giving way, recurvatum, and poor quad function.

13.3.2   Physical Exam

While physical exam findings such as varus or valgus thrust during gait or gross sagittal subluxation on exam may be easier to detect, subtle findings may be more difficult to identify, particularly if the patient is guarding [5]. In full extension the knee may feel stable to varus and valgus stress; however a tight posterior capsule can act as a coronal stabilizer. The knee should also be examined at 30° to isolate the collateral ligaments and at 90° to assess anterior-posterior translation. This is best done with the patient sitting over the edge of the bed with the knee hanging from the table. Patellar tracking abnormalities should also be noted as these can be suggestive of component malrotation.

13.3.3   Radiographs

Careful radiographic analysis can also help identify potential contributing factors. If initial preoperative radiographs are available, they should be examined for significant mechanical axis abnormalities and anatomic deformity as well as increased posterior condylar offset that may have been resected during surgery. Postoperative radiographs including AP, lateral, merchant, and 3 ft standing views should be examined for joint space asymmetry, polyethylene insert size, implant-bone over or undercoverage, patellar tilt, and mechanical axis correction. Stress views are also helpful in delineating varus-valgus instability (AP view) or anterior/posterior instability (lateral view).

13.3.4   Other Tests

Infection should be ruled out in this patient population, oftentimes presenting pain, warmth, and recurrent effusions. It is not unusual that numerous aspirations of the joint due to recurrent effusions have been performed. Multiple aseptic aspirations of recurrent bloody effusions should be an additional clinical insight into possible ligamentous instability etiology of the patient's complaints [6]. Routine inflammatory markers should be assessed in conjunction with aspiration results. If there is suspicion for component malrotation resulting in ligamentous instability, CT scans have been shown to be helpful to identify such abnormalities; however the intra- and interobserver reliability has been variable [7]. CT scan should include the hip joint to assess rotational alignment of the implant in relation to the femoral axis. Full-length standing films can also help diagnose mechanical alignment abnormalities or unrecognized femoral or tibial deformities at the index procedure that may have led to incorrect implant positioning.

13.4   Management

After consideration of both clinical history and physical exam at presentation, a working diagnosis of medial flexion coronal instability in flexion and AP flexion instability (sagittal) was made. Preoperative planning included insurance of implant availability which included constrained components with associated augments compatible with the current implant. Canal reamers and appropriate equipment for component removal including a microsagittal saw, osteotomes, and an available burr were also available.

The previous midline incision was used and extended proximally into native tissue to establish a recognizable tissue dissection plane. A midline parapatellar arthrotomy was carried out and the joint fluid that was encountered was sent for culture. Tissue specimens that were taken from multiple sites and sent to pathology returned intraoperatively with <5 PMNs per high power field in all samples. Intra-articular scar formation was meticulously excised from the medial and lateral gutters and the patellar inversion technique [8] was used for exposure. This technique is our preferred initial exposure and has been shown to provide adequate exposure in >95 % of cases in one study of 420 knee revisions. This involves early lateral retinacular release followed by subperiosteal elevation of the medial ligamentous sleeve while gradually externally rotating the tibia, extending to the posteromedial corner. The rotating platform polyethylene insert was removed with an osteotome after anterior dislocation of the tibia and was inspected for asymmetric as well as backside wear. Attention was then turned to the tibial component which was well fixed and noted to be in appropriate external rotation with regard to the tibial tubercle. At this point the flexion and extension gaps were examined with a tensioning device. The extension gaps were noted to be symmetric; however the flexion gap revealed excessive lateral opening upon tensioning (Fig. 13.2). Based on the tibial component, which was measured to be neutral to the mechanical/anatomic

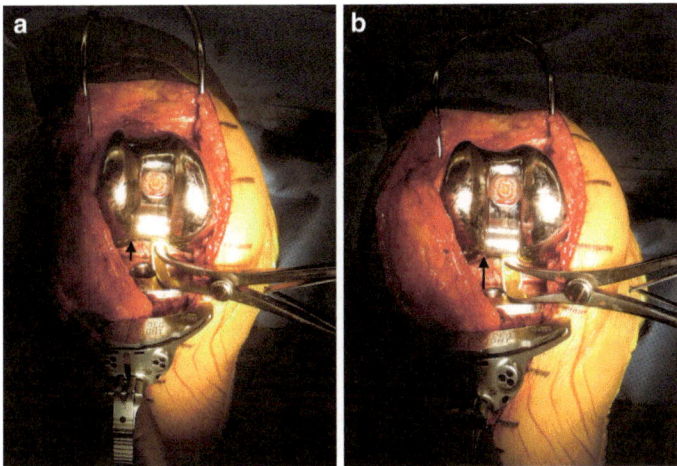

Fig. 13.2. Intraoperative demonstration of ligamentous instability with (**a**) having no tension followed by (**b**) exhibiting lateral opening upon tensioning of the medial and lateral soft tissues.

axis of the tibia, the femoral component was noted to be in approximately 8° of internal rotation while under tension (Fig. 13.3). At this point the decision was made to proceed with femoral revision.

A microsagittal saw was used to disrupt the implant-cement interface in order to conserve as much native bone as possible. A combination of a thin ¼ inch osteotome and the microsagittal saw was used at the chamfer cuts and the distal femur followed by disimpaction of the femur with relatively minimal bone loss. The femoral canal was then reamed sequentially and a 5° distal femoral cut was carried out. At this point a 4 in 1 cutting guide was placed and rotation was set based on the epicondyles and our flexion gap. We noted bone loss both posteriorly and distally and determined the need for corresponding augments to maximize bone-implant contact. Larger augments were placed posterolaterally in order to increase external rotation of the femoral component. The flexion and extension gaps were noted to be equal,

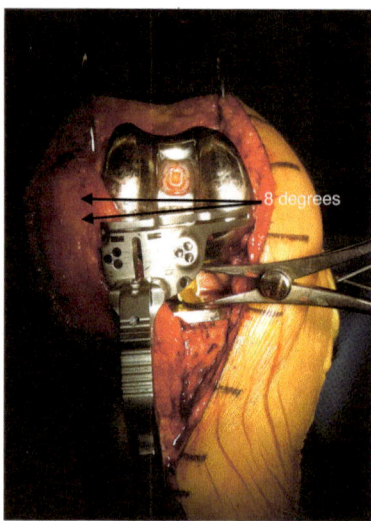

Fig. 13.3. Intraoperative demonstration of improper rotational alignment of the femoral component with internal rotation of approximately 8°.

eliminating the need to posteriorize the femur and a 12.5 mm polyethylene trial was inserted. The knee was stressed at 0, 30, and 90° and deemed stable both in the coronal and sagittal planes. There was noted to be less than 5 mm anterior-posterior shuck at 90° of flexion and there was no gapping with varus/valgus stress in full extension. The synovial scar tissue surrounding the patella was completely debrided and there was no significant wear noted. An osteotome was placed between the bone-implant interface and there was no loosening noted. At 90° of flexion there was mild residual lateral tilt noted and a lateral release was performed, after which the patella tracked well with a no thumbs technique. Antibiotic impregnated cement was mixed on the back table and the femoral implant was cemented in place using a third generation cementing technique. The trial polyethylene was placed and axial pressure was placed on the leg until the cement was dry. The flexion and extension gaps were once again verified and a 12.5 mm polyethylene was seated. Two medium Hemovac drains were placed and the arthrotomy was closed followed by skin closure.

13.5 Outcome

At most recent follow-up visit 2 years following the revision procedure, the patient states that he has increased his activity level and requires no assist devices for ambulation. Patient describes some occasional crepitus around the patella but otherwise no complaints. He denies any further symptoms of instability or giving way and has no difficulty navigating stairs. Examination shows range of motion from 0 to 120° and stable in both coronal and sagittal planes through the full arc of motion. Postoperative radiographs at 3 months are shown in Fig. 13.4.

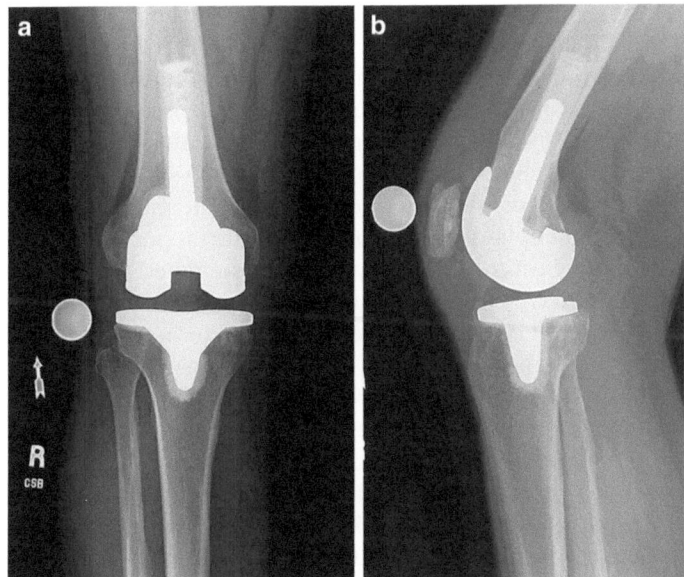

FIG. 13.4. Postoperative AP (**a**) and lateral (**b**) radiographs with new femoral prosthesis and balancing of the soft tissues.

13.6   Management of Ligamentous Instability

It is essential to identify the type of instability that is present before an appropriate preoperative plan can be formulated. There are several etiologies to consider which include component malposition, inadequate restoration of the mechanical axis, ligamentous insufficiency from any cause, and imbalance of flexion-extension gaps. Differing combinations of these can result in three planes of instability to consider: varus-valgus, anterior-posterior(flexion), and global.

Posterior substituting implants introduce constraint in the anterior-posterior plane and can be considered in isolated sagittal instability, specifically in cases where a previous cruciate retaining design was used with subsequent flexion instability. If further stability is required in the coronal plane, additional constraint is achieved using a varus-valgus constrained insert (VVC) which most companies manufacture. This provides both coronal and sagittal restraint as well as partial axial stability by using a taller, wider post and a deeper femoral box. It is important to determine implant specific post/box sizes as these can differ between companies. As constraint increases, so do the forces which are transmitted through the implant-bone interface. In one study, these contact forces were increased 20–60 % compared to a posterior stabilized design [9]. The addition of a stemmed implant can help redistribute a portion of the excess force into the diaphysis. While stemmed constrained implants have been shown to have successful midterm follow-up [10, 11], they have been to found to have drawbacks including pain at the distal tip of the implant [12] and are difficult to remove if future surgery is needed. Currently there has been data suggest a stem may not be needed in a primary knee setting [13]; however this has not been studied in knee revisions where bone stock is often weakened. Thus in the revision setting in which additional constraint is used, a stemmed implant is still recommended. If a constrained insert still does not provide adequate stability, the final option is a rotating hinge. While these have inherent risks such as infection, fracture, and increased loosening, modern implants have been shown to have moderate clinical success [14] and often are the only viable reconstructive option in some cases.

Prior to surgery, constraint options should be considered and availability confirmed with the implant manufacturer. To minimize implant-interface contact stresses, the least amount of constraint should be used [15]. As cruciate retaining implants represent the least constraint in total knee design, these are rarely used in the revision setting.

13.6.1   Flexion Instability

Instability in the anterior-posterior (or sagittal) plane often occurs from a flexion-extension mismatch resulting in a loose flexion gap. This situation can also arise in cruciate retaining prostheses that develop attritional rupture of the native PCL. While the latter can often be corrected with a cruciate substituting insert with a possible upsized insert if needed, the former situation often requires revision of the femoral component. If the joint line is already elevated, the preferred strategy involves addressing the flexion gap by increasing the femoral component size, using a posterior shifted adaptor, and/or using additional posterior augments. A common mistake is to simply increase the polyethylene insert size; however this will often lead to a flexion contracture postoperatively.

13.6.2   Coronal Instability

Varus-valgus (or coronal) instability can be broken down into three categories: extension, flexion, and mid-flexion. Extension instability usually involves imbalance of the collateral ligaments which can be appreciated on physical exam as well as radiographs showing asymmetry of the joint spaces. Often this is the result of incomplete or under release of the concave side and failure to catch up with the convex side during the index procedure. In these cases, further soft tissue release on the concave side may provide sufficient balance to the knee and typically a thicker poly insert is required. A VVC insert is often the poly implant of choice as sufficient balance of the soft tissues throughout the range of motion can be quite difficult in such revisions and may alter the overall flexion gap with manipulation of the extension gap.

Flexion and particularly mid-flexion coronal instability are often more difficult to diagnose and can involve femoral malrotation and/or elements of collateral ligament incompetence. If femoral malrotation is present, there is often symmetry seen in the merchant view of the patellofemoral joint with concomitant patella maltracking. This often can occur from failure to appropriately balance soft tissue at the initial operation or posterior condylar resection that leads to an asymmetric gap in flexion. It has been shown that creating an equal flexion space improves motion and is associated with less postoperative tibial pain [16]. Thus the goal is to achieve a rectangular gap at the time of revision. This is achieved using the flexion gap to determine rotation of the femoral component and if posterior condylar bone loss is present, using augments to provide condylar support in the appropriately determined rotation. If further stability is required, a VVC implant can also be used.

13.6.3   Global Instability

Global instability often presents with frank dislocation or gross multiplanar instability and often is more difficult to manage. Incompetent or nonexistent collateral ligaments may lead to gross multiplanar instability with numerous potential causes. This instability may be directly related to severe preoperative deformity prior to the index procedure never fully addressed, iatrogenic soft tissue injury during the index procedure, or progressive soft tissue laxity. In these cases a rotating hinge prosthesis can be considered and often required to get appropriate stability and function from the revised construct. Primary indications for use of a hinged construct include severe distal femoral bone loss or an infinite flexion gap in which equilibration to the extension gap is not possible.

The goal of revision knee surgery in any of these cases is to restore a mechanically stable, balanced, functional knee. If the specific etiology can be identified prior to surgery, operative efforts will likely be more successful and reproducible outcomes.

13.7 Clinical Pearls/Pitfalls

- Instability following total knee arthroplasty is a common mode of failure and a thorough history and careful physical exam are both crucial to proper management.
- Identifying the mode of instability prior to surgery is necessary for successful surgical outcome.
- As a general rule, the least constraint possible to allow for a stable knee arthroplasty should be utilized.
- Use more than one bony landmark to confirm femoral rotation.
- Elevated suspicion for ligamentous instability with recurrent bloody effusions [6].
- Lateral patella tilt often a sign of femoral or tibial component malrotation.
- CT scan may help assess femoral and tibial component malposition particularly in regard to rotation.
- Constraint is not necessarily required for every revision for ligamentous instability; however equilibration of medial and lateral soft tissue tension may not always be possible and thus necessitate higher constraint within the construct.

References

1. Hernandez-Vaquero D, Sandoval-Garcia MA. Hinged total knee arthroplasty in the presence of ligamentous deficiency. Clin Orthop Relat Res. 2010;468:1248–53.
2. Rose PS, Johnson CA, Hungerford DS, McFarland EG. Total knee arthroplasty in Ehlers-Danlos Syndrome. J Arthroplasty. 2004;19:190–6.
3. Vince KG, Abdeen A, Sugimori T. The unstable total knee arthroplasty: causes and cures. J Arthroplasty. 2006;21:44–9.

4. Fehring TK, Valadie AL. Knee instability after total knee arthroplasty. Clin Orthop Relat Res. 1994;299:157–62.
5. Browne JA, Parratte S, Pagnano MW. Instability in total knee arthroplasty. In: Norman Scott W, editor. Insall and Scott surgery of the knee. 5th ed. Philadelphia: Elsevier; 2011. p. 1359–66.
6. Raab GE, Fehring TK, Odum SM, Mason JB, Griffin WL. Aspiration as an aid to the diagnosis of prosthetic knee instability. Orthopedics. 2009;32(5):318.
7. Konigsberg B, Hess R, Hartman C, Smith L, Garvin KL. Inter- and intraobserver reliability of two-dimensional CT scan for total knee arthroplasty for component malrotation. Clin Orthop Relat Res. 2014;472:212–7.
8. Fehring TK, Odum S, Griffin WL, Mason JB. Patella inversion method for exposure in revision total knee arthroplasty. J Arthroplasty. 2002;17:101–4.
9. Rawlinson JL, Peters LE, Campbell DA, Windsor R, Wright TM, Bartel DL. Cancellous bone strains indicate efficacy of stem augments in constrained condylar knees. Clin Orthop Relat Res. 2005;440:107–16.
10. Haas SB, Insall JN, Montgomery III W, Windsor RE. Revision total knee arthroplasty with use of modular components with stems inserted without cement. J Bone Joint Surg Am. 1995;11:1700–7.
11. Lachiewicz PF, Falatyn SP. Clinical and radiographic results of the total condylar III and constrained condylar total knee arthroplasty. J Arthroplasty. 1996;8:916–22.
12. Barrack RL, Rorabeck C, Burt M, Sawhney J. 1999, Pain at the end of the stem after revision total knee arthroplasty. Clin Orthop Relat Res. 1999;367:216.
13. Nam D, Umunna BN, Cross MB, Reinhardt KR, Duggal S, Cornell CN. Clinical results and failure mechanisms of a nonmodular constrained knee without stem extensions. HSS J. 2012;8:96–102.
14. Pour AE, Parvizi J, Slenker N, Purtill JJ, Sharkey PF. Rotating hinged total knee replacement: use with caution. JBJS. 2007;89:1735–41.
15. Lombardi Jr AV, Berend KR. Posterior cruciate ligament-retaining, posterior stabilized, and varus/valgus posterior stabilized constrained articulations in total knee arthroplasty. Instr Course Lect. 2006;55:419–27.
16. Laskin RS. Flexion space configuration in total knee arthroplasty. J Arthroplasty. 1995;10:657–60.

Index

© Springer International Publishing Switzerland 2015   169
B.D. Springer and B.M. Curtin (eds.), *Complex Primary
and Revision Total Knee Arthroplasty: A Clinical Casebook*,
DOI 10.1007/978-3-319-18350-3